PASTEST POCKET SERIES
FOR MRCP PART 1

D1138258

BOOK 3
MCQs
IN
GASTROENTEROLOGY,
ENDOCRINOLOGY
AND
RENAL MEDICINE

Edited by Richard L. Hawkins MBBS FRCS

Authors: Stephen L. Grainger MD MRCP
David G. Maxton MD MRCP
St Thomas' Hospital,
London.

Gareth Williams MA MD MRCP
Hammersmith Hospital,
London.

Ian Barton MA MRCP
Lucilla Poston PhD
St Thomas' Hospital,
London.

PASTEST

© 1987 PASTEST
Rankin House, Parkgate Estate,
Knutsford, Cheshire. WA16 8DX

First printed 1987
Reprinted 1988
Reprinted 1989
Reprinted 1991
Reprinted 1993

A catalogue record for this book is available from the British Library.

ISBN: 0 906896 23 1

Text prepared by Turner Associates, Knutsford, Cheshire.
Phototypeset by Communitype, Leicester
Printed by Martins The Printers, Berwick on Tweed

CONTENTS

Answers and teaching explanations
are on the back of each question page

INTRODUCTION

With more than twelve years of experience in postgraduate medical education to draw on, PASTEST have commissioned a series of reasonably priced MCQ books under the editorial mantle of Dr Richard Hawkins.

There is no better way to revise for the MRCP Part I examination than by answering good quality MCQs. These books, however, provide an additional dimension. The MCQs have been deliberately broken down by specialty and a self-assessment chart provided for each so that doctors can identify their strengths and weaknesses and plan their revision accordingly.

A significant number of questions in the MRCP Part I examination are devoted to Gastroenterology, Endocrinology and Renal Medicine. This book provides approximately 34 representative questions from each specialty, with each question accompanied by a clear and simple explanatory answer. A strong emphasis on physiology, basic sciences and pharmacology has been included since the modern examination places such importance on these aspects.

The membership examination at present consists of sixty questions, each with a stem and five related questions: a total of 300 possible correct responses. Each correct response is awarded +1, each incorrect one -1, with no marks being awarded if the question is answered 'Don't know'. As in all examinations, proper technique can make the difference between a 'pass' and a 'bare fail'.

What, then, is the best approach? Firstly, the question stem must be read very carefully. Failure to notice a negative statement could result in a score of -5. In a 'close marked' examination this could quite easily be the difference between a pass and a fail. Secondly, the keywords used in MCQs should be identified: always/commonly/frequently/recognised/may/never, and so on. Each has a distinctly different meaning, thus: 'jaundice is a frequent complication of infectious mononucleosis' (false), whereas: 'jaundice may complicate infectious mononucleosis' (true). Beware of always and never.

Finally, answer those questions that you think you have a greater than 50% chance of getting correct. Thus, while leaving out questions in which you would be guessing (because in these you are likely to score 0 overall), do attempt those which you think you know something about; it is worth backing a hunch. Although your 'hit rate' will not be as high for these as for those questions for which you think you know the answer, overall you will score positively. Candidates do fail because they do not attempt enough questions, and it is worth remembering that even some of those answers that you are confident about may, in fact, be wrong.

Time for revision is often at a premium because preparation has to be done at the same time as a busy medical SHO job. A few general tips may be useful:

1. Do not read systematically through large medical textbooks, but rather base your revision around multiple choice questions. The self-assessment charts provided in this book may be helpful here. Direct further reading of standard texts to those areas in which you are scoring low marks, in other words use these MCQs to identify 'blind spots' in your knowledge.

2. Make cards for those questions which come up frequently (such as modes of inheritance) and learn these.

3. A good course is probably worth the investment and your employer may be able to assist with the funding for this, if one is not provided at your hospital.

4. Aim to start your revision in good time and be sure you have time to cover most topics.

Cut-out self-assessment charts are included in this book so that you can record your answers to each MCQ as you work steadily through the questions. In order to give yourself a realistic time limit, do not spend more than 2 ½ minutes on any one question. Some people may prefer to indicate their answers directly on the question pages in the spaces provided and then to transfer these answers on to the self-assessment charts. You can then correct your own answers against the answers given in the book and can calculate your total score in each section. By indicating clearly each item that you answered incorrectly you can then read the explanation provided and refer to a standard textbook for further revision on that topic.

Encyclopaedic specialist reference books are perhaps best avoided during preparation, only to be used for verification of detail. However in the fields of gastroenterology, endocrinology and renal medicine the following titles may be helpful:

Elias and Hawkins. **Lecture Notes on Gastroenterology**. Blackwell.
Thompson, R. **Lecture Notes on the Liver**. Blackwell.
Wilson and Foster. **Williams Textbook of Endocrinology** (7th edition). Saunders.
Wardener, H.E.de. **The Kidney**. Churchill Livingstone.

GASTROENTEROLOGY SELF-ASSESSMENT CHART

Please use 2B PENCIL only. Rub out all errors thoroughly.
Mark lozenges like ➖ NOT like this ⌀ ⌀ ⌀

T ⬤ = TRUE   F ⬤ = FALSE   DK ⬤ = DON'T KNOW

	A	B	C	D	E			A	B	C	D	E
1	T / F / DK	T / F / DK	T / F / DK	T / F / DK	T / F / DK		16	T / F / DK	T / F / DK	T / F / DK	T / F / DK	T / F / DK
2	T / F / DK	T / F / DK	T / F / DK	T / F / DK	T / F / DK		17	T / F / DK	T / F / DK	T / F / DK	T / F / DK	T / F / DK
3	T / F / DK	T / F / DK	T / F / DK	T / F / DK	T / F / DK		18	T / F / DK	T / F / DK	T / F / DK	T / F / DK	T / F / DK
4	T / F / DK	T / F / DK	T / F / DK	T / F / DK	T / F / DK		19	T / F / DK	T / F / DK	T / F / DK	T / F / DK	T / F / DK
5	T / F / DK	T / F / DK	T / F / DK	T / F / DK	T / F / DK		20	T / F / DK	T / F / DK	T / F / DK	T / F / DK	T / F / DK
6	T / F / DK	T / F / DK	T / F / DK	T / F / DK	T / F / DK		21	T / F / DK	T / F / DK	T / F / DK	T / F / DK	T / F / DK
7	T / F / DK	T / F / DK	T / F / DK	T / F / DK	T / F / DK		22	T / F / DK	T / F / DK	T / F / DK	T / F / DK	T / F / DK
8	T / F / DK	T / F / DK	T / F / DK	T / F / DK	T / F / DK		23	T / F / DK	T / F / DK	T / F / DK	T / F / DK	T / F / DK
9	T / F / DK	T / F / DK	T / F / DK	T / F / DK	T / F / DK		24	T / F / DK	T / F / DK	T / F / DK	T / F / DK	T / F / DK
10	T / F / DK	T / F / DK	T / F / DK	T / F / DK	T / F / DK		25	T / F / DK	T / F / DK	T / F / DK	T / F / DK	T / F / DK
11	T / F / DK	T / F / DK	T / F / DK	T / F / DK	T / F / DK		26	T / F / DK	T / F / DK	T / F / DK	T / F / DK	T / F / DK
12	T / F / DK	T / F / DK	T / F / DK	T / F / DK	T / F / DK		27	T / F / DK	T / F / DK	T / F / DK	T / F / DK	T / F / DK
13	T / F / DK	T / F / DK	T / F / DK	T / F / DK	T / F / DK		28	T / F / DK	T / F / DK	T / F / DK	T / F / DK	T / F / DK
14	T / F / DK	T / F / DK	T / F / DK	T / F / DK	T / F / DK		29	T / F / DK	T / F / DK	T / F / DK	T / F / DK	T / F / DK
15	T / F / DK	T / F / DK	T / F / DK	T / F / DK	T / F / DK		30	T / F / DK	T / F / DK	T / F / DK	T / F / DK	T / F / DK

	A	B	C	D	E			A	B	C	D	E
31	T ○	T ○	T ○	T ○	T ○		33	T ○	T ○	T ○	T ○	T ○
	F ○	F ○	F ○	F ○	F ○			F ○	F ○	F ○	F ○	F ○
	DK ○	DK ○	DK ○	DK ○	DK ○			DK ○	DK ○	DK ○	DK ○	DK ○
32	T ○	T ○	T ○	T ○	T ○							
	F ○	F ○	F ○	F ○	F ○							
	DK ○	DK ○	DK ○	DK ○	DK ○							

CORRECT ANSWERS (+1) = _____

INCORRECT ANSWERS (−1) = _____

DON'T KNOW (0) _____

TOTAL SCORE: _____

ENDOCRINOLOGY
SELF-ASSESSMENT CHART

	A	B	C	D	E			A	B	C	D	E
34	T ○	T ○	T ○	T ○	T ○		45	T ○	T ○	T ○	T ○	T ○
	F ○	F ○	F ○	F ○	F ○			F ○	F ○	F ○	F ○	F ○
	DK ○	DK ○	DK ○	DK ○	DK ○			DK ○	DK ○	DK ○	DK ○	DK ○
35	T ○	T ○	T ○	T ○	T ○		46	T ○	T ○	T ○	T ○	T ○
	F ○	F ○	F ○	F ○	F ○			F ○	F ○	F ○	F ○	F ○
	DK ○	DK ○	DK ○	DK ○	DK ○			DK ○	DK ○	DK ○	DK ○	DK ○
36	T ○	T ○	T ○	T ○	T ○		47	T ○	T ○	T ○	T ○	T ○
	F ○	F ○	F ○	F ○	F ○			F ○	F ○	F ○	F ○	F ○
	DK ○	DK ○	DK ○	DK ○	DK ○			DK ○	DK ○	DK ○	DK ○	DK ○
37	T ○	T ○	T ○	T ○	T ○		48	T ○	T ○	T ○	T ○	T ○
	F ○	F ○	F ○	F ○	F ○			F ○	F ○	F ○	F ○	F ○
	DK ○	DK ○	DK ○	DK ○	DK ○			DK ○	DK ○	DK ○	DK ○	DK ○
38	T ○	T ○	T ○	T ○	T ○		49	T ○	T ○	T ○	T ○	T ○
	F ○	F ○	F ○	F ○	F ○			F ○	F ○	F ○	F ○	F ○
	DK ○	DK ○	DK ○	DK ○	DK ○			DK ○	DK ○	DK ○	DK ○	DK ○
39	T ○	T ○	T ○	T ○	T ○		50	T ○	T ○	T ○	T ○	T ○
	F ○	F ○	F ○	F ○	F ○			F ○	F ○	F ○	F ○	F ○
	DK ○	DK ○	DK ○	DK ○	DK ○			DK ○	DK ○	DK ○	DK ○	DK ○
40	T ○	T ○	T ○	T ○	T ○		51	T ○	T ○	T ○	T ○	T ○
	F ○	F ○	F ○	F ○	F ○			F ○	F ○	F ○	F ○	F ○
	DK ○	DK ○	DK ○	DK ○	DK ○			DK ○	DK ○	DK ○	DK ○	DK ○
41	T ○	T ○	T ○	T ○	T ○		52	T ○	T ○	T ○	T ○	T ○
	F ○	F ○	F ○	F ○	F ○			F ○	F ○	F ○	F ○	F ○
	DK ○	DK ○	DK ○	DK ○	DK ○			DK ○	DK ○	DK ○	DK ○	DK ○
42	T ○	T ○	T ○	T ○	T ○		53	T ○	T ○	T ○	T ○	T ○
	F ○	F ○	F ○	F ○	F ○			F ○	F ○	F ○	F ○	F ○
	DK ○	DK ○	DK ○	DK ○	DK ○			DK ○	DK ○	DK ○	DK ○	DK ○
43	T ○	T ○	T ○	T ○	T ○		54	T ○	T ○	T ○	T ○	T ○
	F ○	F ○	F ○	F ○	F ○			F ○	F ○	F ○	F ○	F ○
	DK ○	DK ○	DK ○	DK ○	DK ○			DK ○	DK ○	DK ○	DK ○	DK ○
44	T ○	T ○	T ○	T ○	T ○		55	T ○	T ○	T ○	T ○	T ○
	F ○	F ○	F ○	F ○	F ○			F ○	F ○	F ○	F ○	F ○
	DK ○	DK ○	DK ○	DK ○	DK ○			DK ○	DK ○	DK ○	DK ○	DK ○

	A	B	C	D	E		A	B	C	D	E
56	T / F / DK	T / F / DK	T / F / DK	T / F / DK	T / F / DK	62	T / F / DK	T / F / DK	T / F / DK	T / F / DK	T / F / DK
57	T / F / DK	T / F / DK	T / F / DK	T / F / DK	T / F / DK	63	T / F / DK	T / F / DK	T / F / DK	T / F / DK	T / F / DK
58	T / F / DK	T / F / DK	T / F / DK	T / F / DK	T / F / DK	64	T / F / DK	T / F / DK	T / F / DK	T / F / DK	T / F / DK
59	T / F / DK	T / F / DK	T / F / DK	T / F / DK	T / F / DK	65	T / F / DK	T / F / DK	T / F / DK	T / F / DK	T / F / DK
60	T / F / DK	T / F / DK	T / F / DK	T / F / DK	T / F / DK	66	T / F / DK	T / F / DK	T / F / DK	T / F / DK	T / F / DK
61	T / F / DK	T / F / DK	T / F / DK	T / F / DK	T / F / DK						

CORRECT ANSWERS (+1) =

INCORRECT ANSWERS (−1) =

DON'T KNOW (0) _____

TOTAL SCORE: _____

RENAL MEDICINE SELF-ASSESSMENT CHART

	A	B	C	D	E		A	B	C	D	E
67	T / F / DK	T / F / DK	T / F / DK	T / F / DK	T / F / DK	72	T / F / DK	T / F / DK	T / F / DK	T / F / DK	T / F / DK
68	T / F / DK	T / F / DK	T / F / DK	T / F / DK	T / F / DK	73	T / F / DK	T / F / DK	T / F / DK	T / F / DK	T / F / DK
69	T / F / DK	T / F / DK	T / F / DK	T / F / DK	T / F / DK	74	T / F / DK	T / F / DK	T / F / DK	T / F / DK	T / F / DK
70	T / F / DK	T / F / DK	T / F / DK	T / F / DK	T / F / DK	75	T / F / DK	T / F / DK	T / F / DK	T / F / DK	T / F / DK
71	T / F / DK	T / F / DK	T / F / DK	T / F / DK	T / F / DK	76	T / F / DK	T / F / DK	T / F / DK	T / F / DK	T / F / DK

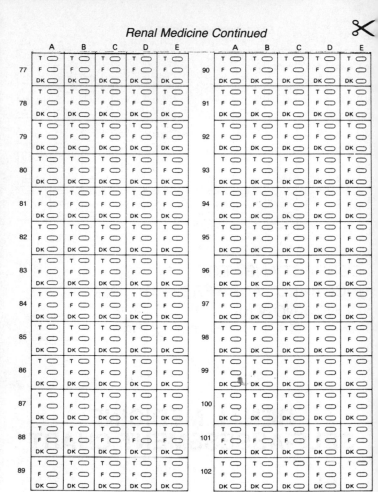

CORRECT ANSWERS (+1) =

INCORRECT ANSWERS (−1) =

DON'T KNOW (0) _____

TOTAL SCORE: _____

X

GASTROENTEROLOGY

Indicate your answers by putting T (True), F (False) or D (Don't know) in the spaces provided.

1. Reflux oesophagitis
A is characterised by increased oesophageal clearance of refluxed material
B is associated with Barrett's oesophagus
C occurs commonly in systemic sclerosis
D can be reliably diagnosed by histology
E can be treated with anticholinergic drugs

Your answers: A.........B.........C.........D.........E.........

2. Bilirubin
A is entirely formed from haemoglobin breakdown
B before liver conjugation is transported in the blood bound to serum albumin
C in the blood of normal subjects is predominantly conjugated
D when conjugated is water soluble
E is metabolised to urobilinogen by gut bacterial action

Your answers: A.........B.........C.........D.........E.........

3. Perforation of the oesophagus
A may occur during endoscopic dilatation
B after retching usually occurs in the upper oesophagus
C is characterised by surgical emphysema
D is associated with pleural effusions
E occurring spontaneously should be managed conservatively

Your answers: A.........B.........C.........D.........E.........

Answers overleaf

ANSWERS AND EXPLANATIONS

1. **B C**

   Patients with oesophagitis suffer frequent acid reflux, have reduced oesophageal clearance and may have reduced mucosal resistance. Oesophagitis is associated with hiatus hernia, pregnancy, systemic sclerosis and irritable bowel syndrome, and may follow the successful treatment of achalasia. Diagnosis is usually from the history and endoscopy best demonstrates the accompanying inflammation. Histology is of little value but 24 hr oesophageal pH measurement may be helpful. Complications include oesophageal stricture and Barrett's oesophagus, which is a pre-malignant condition. Treatment is unsatisfactory, but anticholinergics should be avoided since they reduce oesophageal motility and the tone of the lower oesophageal sphincter.

2. **B D E**

   Bilirubin is formed from haem, but only 70% from haemoglobin, the remainder coming from non-erythroid haem and haemoproteins often in the liver. Unconjugated bilirubin, which makes up virtually all the serum bilirubin in normal subjects, is water insoluble, and therefore is transported to the liver bound to serum albumin. In the liver it is conjugated with glucuronic acid to increase water solubility and facilitate excretion. In the gut it is metabolised by gut bacteria to urobilinogen which undergoes an enterohepatic circulation.

3. **A C D**

   Oesophageal perforation may be spontaneous or secondary to trauma from a foreign body or during endoscopy. Spontaneous perforation usually occurs after forceful retching and the tear is usually in the lower oesophagus. Patients present with acute severe chest pain, similar to myocardial infarction and fever, dyspnoea, shock, pleural effusion, and pneumothorax. Surgical emphysema in the neck may be present. Radiography may reveal mediastinal air and air in the tissue planes of the neck. Treatment is surgical. Endoscopic perforation usually occurs in elderly patients following dilatation. Many can be managed conservatively with intravenous antibiotics, nil by mouth and nutritional support.

4. Systemic sclerosis of the gastrointestinal tract
A most commonly affects the oesophagus
B is associated with primary biliary cirrhosis
C causes narrowing of the small intestinal lumen
D may produce diarrhoea responding to antibiotic therapy
E is a recognised cause of steatorrhoea

Your answers: A.........B.........C.........D.........E.........

5. In the normal liver
A a portal tract contains a branch of the portal vein, hepatic arteriole and bile ductule
B after feeding the portal vein provides 35-40% of total liver blood flow
C hepatocytes make up 60-70% of the total liver cell mass
D the hepatic veins drain directly into the inferior vena cava
E there are no reticulo-endothelial cells

Your answers: A.........B.........C.........D.........E.........

6. H₂ antagonists
A may cause impotence
B increase plasma gastrin levels
C are contraindicated in renal failure
D are cytoprotective
E decrease both basal and stimulated acid secretion

Your answers: A.........B.........C.........D.........E.........

Answers overleaf

4. A B D E

The gastrointestinal tract is frequently affected in systemic sclerosis with the oesophagus being involved in up to 80% of patients. Abnormalities are best seen by manometry and include low resting oesophageal pressure and non-progressive contractions. Symptoms include heartburn, dysphagia for liquids and solids and pulmonary aspiration on lying down. Stomach involvement is rare, but systemic sclerosis causes dilatation and stasis of the small intestine and delayed transit. Abdominal pain, distension, diarrhoea and steatorrhoea, which is probably due to bacterial overgrowth, may occur. Colonic symptoms are uncommon. Systemic sclerosis is associated with autoimmune disease such as primary biliary cirrhosis and the C.R.E.S.T. syndrome.

5. A C D

The normal liver weighs 1.2-1.5 kg, has a large right and smaller left lobe and a dual blood supply. One third of the total liver blood flow comes from the coeliac axis via the hepatic artery. The remainder is drained from the intestine and the spleen via the portal vein. Post-prandial splanchnic hyperaemia increases the portal vein's contribution to more than 75%. Liver structure is based on the hepatic lobule centred on a tributary of the hepatic vein, which is separated by columns of hepatocytes and sinusoids from the portal tracts. Each tract contains a portal vein radicle, hepatic arteriole and bile ductule. Hepatocytes make up 60-70% of total liver cells. The reticulo-endothelial system is well represented in the liver particularly by the Kupffer cells.

6. A B E

These drugs block the action of histamine on the gastric parietal cell H_2 receptor and therefore reduce basal and stimulated acid and pepsin secretion. They have no clinically useful cytoprotective action to increase mucosal resistance. Serum gastrin levels rise a little in response to the hypochlorhydria. The drugs may be used in renal failure but in a reduced dosage. Cimetidine prolongs the elimination of some drugs, particularly warfarin and phenytoin, by inhibiting hepatic cytochrome P_{450}. Increased prolactin levels, gynaecomastia, impotence, confusion in the elderly, tiredness and diarrhoea have been reported. Ranitidine does not affect the activity of cytochrome P_{450}, nor prolactin secretion. Other side effects are probably comparable.

7. Duodenal ulceration
A relapse occurs in about two thirds of patients within one year after H_2 antagonist treatment
B barium meals produce more 'false-negatives' than endoscopy
C is associated with increased acid secretion
D patients failing to respond to H_2 antagonists require surgery
E tends to be familial

Your answers: A.........B.........C.........D.........E.........

8. Infantile hypertrophic pyloric stenosis
A has an increased familial incidence
B maximum incidence is between 2-3 months of age
C is associated with hypochloraemic acidosis
D is more common in boys
E vomitus may contain blood, but not bile

Your answers: A.........B.........C.........D.........E.........

9. Gastric carcinoma
A incidence in the UK is declining
B is associated with previous surgery to the stomach
C most tumours are palpable on first presentation
D is associated with hyperacidity
E lymph node spread is rare

Your answers: A.........B.........C.........D.........E.........

Answers overleaf

7. A B C E

Duodenal ulcers are more common than gastric ulcers. There is a familial tendency to develop the disease, and many patients have increased acid secretion, especially at night. The investigation of choice is endoscopy since active ulcers may be missed on barium meal particularly if the duodenal bulb is scarred from previous disease. Relapse is very common after acute therapy, more than two thirds recurring within one year. If initial H_2 antagonist therapy fails to heal the ulcer, increased dosage, or alternative therapy with a cytoprotective agent or addition of another antisecretory drug should be tried. Surgery is reserved for complications or persistent ulceration despite continuous drug therapy.

8. A D E

Hypertrophic pyloric stenosis occurs in 3 per 1,000 infants in the UK. Males outnumber females 4:1. There is an increased familial incidence and associations with Turner's syndrome, oesophageal atresia and phenylketonuria. The condition presents with vomiting characteristically between 2-4 weeks of age and rarely after 2 months. Vomitus is not bile- stained, but in 20% contains altered blood. Examination may reveal visible gastric peristalsis and a palpable tumour in the right hypochondrium in addition to signs of weight loss and dehydration. Loss of gastric juice produces a hypochloraemic alkalosis. Anticholinergic drugs may be tried but treatment is usually surgical.

9. A B

The incidence of gastric carcinoma is declining in the UK, although there is a marked geographical variability with increased incidence particularly in Japan. Associations include blood group A, male sex, low socio-economic group and smoking. Predisposing causes include achlorhydria and pernicious anaemia, intestinal metaplasia and previous gastric surgery. Histologically most (95%) are adenocarcinomas and present with abdominal pain, anorexia, gastrointestinal haemorrhage, dysphagia and vomiting. An abdominal mass is palpable only in 33%. Surgery is the treatment of choice, but most have lymph node involvement at the time of surgery. Thus 5 year survival is usually less that 10%.

10. Hirschsprung's disease

A is more common in girls

B occurs commonly distally in the colon

C the affected aganglionic segment is grossly dilated on barium enema

D may be conclusively diagnosed by rectal biopsy

E may be associated with growth retardation

Your answers: A.........B.........C.........D.........E.........

11. Oesophageal carcinoma

A is a complication of achalasia

B adenocarcinomas have a better prognosis than squamous at the same site

C occurs more frequently in patients with coeliac disease

D causing tracheo-oesophageal fistula is a contraindication to insertion of a prosthetic tube

E loss of weight is a prominent feature

Your answers: A.........B.........C.........D.........E.........

12. In ulcerative colitis

A barium enema is the most sensitive indication of disease extent

B rectal sparing is characteristic

C rectal biopsy may be useful in detecting malignant change

D histological change may be mimicked by *Shigella* infection

E may be complicated by constipation

Your answers: A.........B.........C.........D.........E.........

10. B D E

Hirschsprung's disease is due to congenital absence of the myenteric parasympathetic nerve cells in Auerbach's plexus of a segment of the colon. This occurs more commonly distally in the colon, with 30% confined to the rectum and only 10% extending beyond the sigmoid. There is a familial distribution and the disease is commoner in boys. Most cases present in the first week of life with intestinal obstruction, but some patients present much later with chronic constipation, anorexia, failure to thrive and growth retardation. Diagnosis is made by barium enema which demonstrates the narrowed aganglionic segment and may be confirmed by full thickness rectal biopsy showing absence of ganglion cells. Treatment is surgical.

11. A C E

The incidence is rising, perhaps because of the increased ingestion of nitrosamines and alcohol, and also nutritional deficiencies of vitamins and trace elements. Associated conditions include achalasia, coeliac disease, Barrett's oesophagus and the Paterson-Kelly syndrome. Dysphagia initially for solids only and weight loss are prominent early symptoms. Histologically most tumours are squamous carcinomas except in the lower oesophagus. Treatment is either by radical or palliative surgery or by radiotherapy, but prognosis is poor, particularly for adenocarcinomas, with only a 20% 5 year survival. Complications such as total dysphagia or tracheo-bronchial fistula may be treated by endoscopic insertion of a prosthetic tube.

12. C D E

Ulcerative colitis usually begins in the rectum, and extends proximally for a variable extent. The histological changes are limited to the mucosa of the colon but are not pathognomonic since infection by *Shigella*, *Campylobacter* and other bacteria may cause similar changes. Proximal constipation may occur but diarrhoea with rectal bleeding and mucus occur most commonly. Disease extent is best assessed by endoscopy with multiple biopsies rather than by barium enema. There is an increased risk of colorectal cancer, which positively correlates with the duration and extent of the colitis. Surveillance of this group with regular rectal biopsy to detect dysplastic change of the epithelium or colonoscopy is recommended.

13. In irritable bowel syndrome
A nocturnal diarrhoea is a feature
B pain is not necessarily a feature
C there is an association with menstrual disturbance
D defaecation characteristically increases abdominal pain
E onset may be precipitated by intestinal infections

Your answers: A........B.........C.........D.........E.........

14. Bile acids
A are formed in the liver from cholesterol
B are conjugated with taurine and glycine before excretion into bile
C are about 50% reabsorbed from the intestinal lumen
D cannot be metabolised by intestinal bacteria
E are synthesised at up to 10 mg/day in normal individuals

Your answers: A........B.........C.........D.........E.........

15. Pseudomembranous colitis
A typically spares the rectum
B may occur after metronidazole
C is caused by toxin producing *Clostridium difficile*
D is best treated with intravenous vancomycin
E relapse is very uncommon after treatment

Your answers: A........B.........C.........D.........E.........

Answers overleaf

13. B C E

Common symptoms of irritable bowel syndrome include col-
icky abdominal pain anywhere in the abdomen, relief of pain
with defaecation, abdominal distension with bloating and
alternating constipation and diarrhoea. Nocturnal diarrhoea is
rare in this functional disorder. Variants of this syndrome
include patients in whom pain is predominant with little bowel
disturbance, and those who complain of painless diarrhoea,
characteristically in the morning soon after rising. Patients
often complain of upper gastrointestinal symptoms and are
more prone to menstrual disturbance. Onset of the syndrome
following acute infective diarrhoea is usually associated with
short-lived symptoms.

14. A B

Normally 300-500 mg/day of cholesterol are converted in the
liver into cholic and chenodeoxycholic acid. Before secretion
into the bile these primary bile acids are conjugated with
taurine and glycine. Bile acids are strong detergents helping to
maintain cholesterol and bilirubin soluble in bile. 96% of bile
acids are reabsorbed into an enterohepatic circulation from
the small intestine and colon. A proportion of the primary bile
acids are metabolised by intestinal bacteria to the secondary
bile acids, deoxycholic acid and lithocholic acid.

15. B C

Pseudomembranous colitis describes the development of colonic inflammation in association with the use of antimicrobial
drugs. Clindamycin was the antibiotic initially associated with
this condition, but many broad spectrum antibiotics are now
implicated. The cause is infection with a toxin producing strain
of *Clostridium difficile*. Multiple raised yellowish-white plaques
are seen predominantly in the distal colon, although on rare
occasions the rectum is spared. *C. difficile*, but not the toxin,
may be found in the stools of 3% of normal adults and up to
50% of healthy neonates. Treatment is with oral vancomycin,
oral or intravenous metronidazole or oral bacitracin. Relapse
occurs in up to 33% of cases.

16. **Benign gastric ulcers**
    A are usually situated on the greater curvature
    B occur more frequently in patients receiving steroids
    C are more common in men than women
    D are usually multiple
    E are associated with increased acid secretion, especially at
      night

    Your answers: A.........B.........C.........D.........E.........

17. **Folic acid**
    A is absorbed predominantly in the jejunum
    B blood level is reduced in stagnant loop syndrome
    C bioavailability is impaired by cooking
    D body stores are adequate for 3 years
    E is effective treatment for alcohol-induced macrocytosis

    Your answers: A.........B.........C.........D.........E.........

18. **Coeliac disease is characterised by**
    A reduced intestinal lactase activity
    B association with HLA-B8
    C increased polymorphs in the lamina propria
    D reduced villus and crypt length
    E increased incidence of antibodies to casein

    Your answers: A.........B.........C.........D.........E.........

16. **B C**

Benign gastric ulcers are commonest in the 50-60 age group, particularly in men who smoke. Most patients complain of epigastric pain, often at night. Aetiological factors probably include delayed gastric emptying, increased bile reflux and defective mucosal resistance, but excess acid secretion is not present. No association has been shown between benign gastric ulceration and alcohol intake, but steroid therapy doubles the incidence. Most benign gastric ulcers occur on the lesser curve of the stomach or in the prepyloric region. Ulcers are multiple only in about 5% of patients.

17. **A C**

Folic acid is found in liver, nuts and green vegetables but is degraded by cooking. Absorption of the daily requirement of 100-200 μg occurs in the duodenum and jejunum. Body stores are sufficient for four months. Causes of folate malabsorption include coeliac disease, tropical sprue, jejunal and gastric resection, intestinal lymphoma, and drugs particularly methotrexate and sulphasalazine. In stagnant loop syndrome folic acid is synthesised by bacteria and blood concentrations are increased. Alcoholic macrocytosis does not respond to folate supplementation.

18. **A B E**

Coeliac disease has a familial incidence and a geographical variability, the disease being particularly common in the West of Ireland and an association with HLA-B8 and DR3. The aetiology is a sensitivity to gliadin, part of the gluten protein found in wheat, rye and barley. Diagnosis depends on demonstrating villus atrophy, on jejunal biopsy, with reduced villus height but increased crypt depth and increased lymphocytes in the lamina propria and intra-epithelially. Intestinal lactase activity and nutrient absorption are reduced, but permeability increased. Increased plasma levels of antibodies to food products including gliadin and casein occur.

19. Intestinal glucose absorption
  A is a passive process
  B from dietary starch requires prior luminal hydrolysis by pancreatic amylase
  C is sodium-dependent
  D from sucrose requires brush border disaccharidase activity
  E shares a common carrier with galactose

  Your answers: A.........B.........C.........D.........E.........

20. Dietary fat
  A is ingested primarily as cholesterol
  B is absorbed predominantly as free fatty acids and monoglyceride
  C absorption is enhanced by low pH
  D absorption is enhanced by bile salts
  E absorption is predominantly into the portal vein

  Your answers: A.........B.........C.........D.........E.........

21. Dietary protein
  A is hydrolysed in the stomach by pepsin to free amino acids
  B as free amino acids is absorbed by a common transport system
  C absorption is an active process
  D is digested by trypsin and chymotrypsin which are secreted in active form by the pancreas
  E absorption from dipeptides is faster than from constituent amino acids

  Your answers: A.........B.........C.........D.........E.........

Answers overleaf

19. B C D E

Carbohydrate is mostly ingested as starch or the disaccharides sucrose and lactose. Starch is hydrolysed in the lumen by pancreatic amylase to disaccharides and α-limit dextrins. These oligo- and disaccharides are then hydrolysed by specific mucosal enzymes to their constituent monosaccharides, predominantly glucose, galactose and fructose. Glucose and galactose share a common active sodium-dependent pathway while fructose is absorbed independently by facilitated diffusion.

20. B D

70 g of dietary fat is ingested daily predominantly as triglycerides, which are hydrolysed by pancreatic lipase to free fatty acids and monoglycerides before absorption. This process requires firstly emulsification of ingested fat and then the formation of micelles of cholesterol, free fatty acids and monoglycerides. The micelles then break up on the mucosal surface allowing the constituents to diffuse passively into the cell where triglycerides are reformed and pass into the lymphatics. Low pH inactivates pancreatic lipase, while bile acids aid formation of micelles.

21. C E

Dietary protein is initially hydrolysed by pepsin in the stomach to produce polypeptides. These are further hydrolysed in the duodenum and jejunum by pancreatic trypsin, chymotrypsin, elastase and carboxypeptidases to small peptide molecules and free amino acids. These digestive enzymes are secreted in inactive form and require activation by specific splitting of the protein molecule. Free amino acids are actively absorbed by three different group-specific enzymes. Some dipeptides are absorbed intact while others are broken down by mucosal peptidases. Absorption from dipeptides is faster than that from the constituent amino acids.

22. The following statements are true:

A somatostatin inhibits release of most gastrointestinal hormones

B enteroglucagon is the major trophic hormone of the small intestine

C secretin increases biliary secretion and gall bladder emptying

D somatostatin is a peptide produced by the beta cells of the pancreas

E excess vasoactive intestinal polypeptide causes hypokalaemia

Your answers: A.........B.........C.........D.........E.........

23. The following statements are true of sulphasalazine:

A most side effects are due to the 5-amino-salicylic acid moeity

B it may cause headaches

C it is of established value in the maintenance of remission of ulcerative colitis

D it is contraindicated in pregnancy

E it may produce reversible male impotence

Your answers: A.........B.........C.........D.........E.........

24. Recognised gastrointestinal infections in AIDS include

A cytomegalovirus

B *Cryptococcus neoformans*

C herpes simplex virus

D *Pneumocystis carinii*

E atypical mycobacteria

Your answers: A.........B.........C.........D.........E.........

Answers overleaf

22. A B E

Somatostatin is a peptide produced by the D cells of the islets of Langerhans. It inhibits the release of most gastrointestinal hormones and reduces intestinal and liver blood flow. Enteroglucagon is released from the terminal ileum and is probably the major trophic hormone to the gut. Secretin stimulates the production of pancreatic bicarbonate; while cholecystokinin contracts the gall bladder (and other intestinal smooth muscle), and stimulates pancreatic enzyme release. Vasoactive intestinal polypeptide (VIP) in excess produces severe watery diarrhoea with hypokalaemia and acidosis (Verner-Morrison syndrome). Its normal function is as a neurotransmitter.

23. B C

Sulphasalazine was originally synthesised to treat rheumatoid arthritis. It is a combination of 5-amino-salicylic acid (5-ASA) and sulphapyridine linked by a diazo bond, which is split by colonic bacteria. Most side effects are due to sulphapyridine while 5-ASA is the therapeutic moiety. It is of proven value in acute ulcerative colitis and colonic Crohn's disease and in prevention of relapse of ulcerative colitis. It is safe in pregnancy. Side effects include skin rashes, headache, nausea, abnormal liver function tests, haemolysis and a reversible decrease in sperm count, but the drug does not affect potency.

24. A C E

Intestinal infection in the acquired immunodeficiency syndrome is common. In the oesophagus, herpes simplex, *Candida albicans* or cytomegalovirus may be the causative agent. Opportunistic small bowel disease occurs with *Cryptosporidium, Isospora belli*, other sporing protozoa or atypical mycobacterium such as *M. avium intracellulare* mimicking Whipple's disease. Colitis may be due to herpes simplex or cytomegalovirus. Gastrointestinal Kaposi's sarcoma may be the initial presentation of AIDS; *Cryptococcus neoformans* usually causes a meningitis and *Pneumocystis* a pneumonia.

25. In hepatitis B infection

A HB$_s$Ag is present in the serum before clinical jaundice
B the virus is a DNA virus
C materno-fetal transmission is rare
D delta agent superinfection may occur after HB$_s$Ag is cleared from the blood
E active immunisation produces positive antibody response in most recipients

Your answers: A.........B.........C.........D.........E.........

26. Alcohol

A is metabolised by alcohol dehydrogenase
B in excess is associated with constrictive cardiomyopathy
C excess is associated with red cell macrocytosis
D excess causes increased hepatic iron accumulation
E causes feminisation by diminishing pituitary gonadotrophin release

Your answers: A.........B.........C.........D.........E.........

27. The following are causes of neonatal conjugated hyper-bilirubinaemia:

A hereditary fructose intolerance
B α-1 antitrypsin deficiency
C biliary atresia
D haemolytic disease of the newborn
E intravenous nutrition

Your answers: A.........B.........C.........D.........E.........

Answers overleaf

25. A B E

Hepatitis B is caused by a 43 nm DNA virus. Incubation period is 60-160 days and spread is parenterally, by sexual contact, shared needles or materno-fetal perinatal transmission. Hepatitis B surface antigen (HB_sAg) is detected in the serum 3-6 weeks after a primary infection and before clinical jaundice. It is usually cleared within a further 3 months. Active immunisation is effective against hepatitis B infection with over 90% positive response, although lower seroconversion rates occur in homosexuals. Delta agent is an incomplete RNA virus that produces liver disease solely in patients with hepatitis B virus infection since it requires HB_sAg for transfer between liver cells.

26. A C D E

90% of ingested alcohol is metabolised in the liver by the non-microsomal enzyme alcohol dehydrogenase to acetaldehyde which is converted to acetate by aldehyde dehydrogenase. Clinical pointers to alcohol abuse include red cell macrocytosis and the presence of more than three fractured ribs. Hepatic iron content is increased making differentiation from haemochromatosis necessary. Complications include dilated cardiomyopathy, and gynaecomastia and testicular atrophy due to primary gonadal failure, depressed hypothalamic-pituitary function and disturbed hepatic metabolism of oestrogens and gonadotrophins.

27. B C E

Causes of neonatal conjugated hyperbilirubinaemia include generalised bacterial infections, toxoplasmosis, hepatitis B, drugs, intravenous nutrition, galactosaemia, α-1 antitrypsin deficiency and hypothyroidism. Any cause of biliary obstruction including biliary atresia and choledochal cysts also cause conjugated hyperbilirubinaemia. Fructosaemia does not usually cause symptoms until fructose is ingested in the diet commonly at the time of weaning. Haemolytic disease will give an unconjugated hyperbilirubinaemia.

28. In primary biliary cirrhosis

A positive antimitochondrial antibodies occur in over 95% of patients

B pruritus may be the only clinical feature

C centri-zonal necrosis is the characteristic liver histopathology

D liver copper is increased

E there is an association with Sjögren's syndrome

Your answers: A.........B.........C.........D.........E.........

29. In childhood coeliac disease

A a flat small intestinal biopsy is diagnostic

B growth failure is common

C intestinal hypolactasia may occur

D intestinal sugar permeability is decreased

E clinical and histological response is more rapid than in adults

Your answers: A.........B.........C.........D.........E.........

30. Wilson's disease is associated with

A extrapyramidal neurological signs

B excess hepatic iron

C increased serum caeruloplasmin

D Kayser-Fleischer rings

E isolated psychiatric illness

Your answers: A.........B.........C.........D.........E.........

Answers overleaf

28. A B D E

Over 95% of patients with primary biliary cirrhosis have positive serum antimitochondrial antibodies, although they are not specific for primary biliary cirrhosis since positive results occur in some other liver diseases. Excess liver accumulation of copper accompanies the cholestasis, but is not usually sufficient to cause confusion with Wilson's disease. Centri-zonal necrosis is not a feature. Associated conditions include rheumatoid arthritis, scleroderma, Sjógren's syndrome, pancreatic atrophy and renal tubular acidosis.

29. B C

Atrophy of the small intestinal mucosa may accompany gut infections and cows' milk protein allergy in childhood, as well as coeliac disease. Failure to thrive is a common presentation and diarrhoea may not be gross. Mucosal permeability to sugars is increased and hypolactasia occurs because of the damage to the enterocytes. Response to gluten withdrawal is usually rapid but may be delayed.

30. A D E

Wilson's disease is a rare inherited disease of copper metabolism that causes isolated hepatic, neurological or psychiatric disease or a combination of these. Neurological signs are usually extrapyramidal. Biochemical abnormalities include reduced serum caeruloplasmin, increased hepatic copper, and excess urinary copper. Accumulation of copper in the cornea produces Kayser-Fleischer rings in about 50% of patients; such changes also rarely occur in other hepatic conditions that are accompanied by prolonged cholestasis.

1. Oesophageal varices

A may occur without liver disease

B rarely bleed when portal pressure is below 14 mm Hg

C survival after bleeding is independent of the severity of liver disease

D that bleed should be treated by emergency porto-systemic shunting

E accompany raised portal pressure, which is reduced by non-selective beta-blockers

Your answers: A.........B.........C.........D.........E.........

2. Delayed gastric emptying

A occurs in hyperglycaemia

B after vagotomy responds to metoclopramide

C is a feature of the dumping syndrome

D is caused by anti-parkinsonian drugs

E may be detected by a succussion splash

Your answers: A.........B.........C.........D.........E.........

3. In Gilbert's syndrome

A jaundice is exacerbated by fasting

B liver histology is diagnostic

C bilirubinuria occurs

D death before 30 years is frequent

E the incidence of gall stones is increased

Your answers: A.........B.........C.........D.........E.........

Answers overleaf

31. A B E

In portal hypertension portal blood is shunted through col lateral veins into the superior and inferior vena cava via oesophageal, gastric, umbilical and rectal veins. Extra-hepatic (presinusoidal) portal hypertension may occur because of intra-abdominal sepsis, particularly after umbilical vein catheterisation in neonates, or from compression of the portal vein by tumour or in conditions causing splenomegaly. Large varices bleed and these usually accompany portal pressures greater than 14 mm Hg. Emergency endoscopic sclerotherapy is now the treatment of choice to control haemorrhage, but the patient's survival depends on the underlying liver condition. Rebleeding is reduced by non selective beta-blockers, which diminish splanchnic blood flow but sclerotherapy is more effective.

32. A B D E

Hyperglycaemia reduces vagal tone to the stomach and thus slows gastric emptying. Any condition that causes slow gastric emptying (e.g. pyloric stenosis) may be accompanied by a succussion splash. After truncal vagotomy the gastric intrinsic nerves remain intact and still release acetyl choline in response to metoclopramide. Dumping is caused by accelerated emptying of hyperosmolar nutrients into the small intestine. Anti-parkinsonian drugs slow gastric emptying by blocking cholinergic muscarinic receptors or by being dopamine agonists.

33. A

Gilbert's syndrome is a benign, familial, mild unconjugated hyperbilirubinaemia affecting 2-5% of the population, probably inherited as an autosomal dominant. Jaundice is exacerbated by fasting and following intravenous nicotinic acid which has been used as a diagnostic test. Liver histology is normal, the jaundice being due to reduced activity of bilirubin conjugating enzymes. Although erythrocyte survival may be mildly reduced, gall stones are not more frequent. Life expectancy is normal.

ENDOCRINOLOGY

Indicate your answers by putting T (True), F (False) or D (Don't know) in the spaces provided.

34. The close anatomical relations of the pituitary fossa include
  A the cavernous sinus
  B the internal carotid artery
  C the third cranial nerve
  D the sphenoidal sinus
  E the eighth cranial nerve

  Your answers: A.........B.........C.........D.........E.........

35. Craniopharyngioma is commonly associated with
  A intrasellar calcification visible on a plain skull X-ray
  B diabetes insipidus
  C optic atrophy
  D hyperprolactinaemia
  E good response to treatment

  Your answers: A.........B.........C.........D.........E.........

36. Elevated prolactin levels are associated with
  A acromegaly
  B dopaminergic agonists
  C pregnancy
  D metoclopramide
  E external beam radiotherapy treatment of pituitary tumours

  Your answers: A.........B.........C.........D.........E.........

Answers overleaf

34. A B C D

A number of important structures lie close to the pituitary fossa and can be encroached upon by an expanding pituitary tumour. Immediately lateral to the fossa (which does not have bony lateral walls) lies the cavernous sinus, through which runs the sixth cranial nerve. The third, fourth and upper two divisions of the fifth cranial nerves lie in the lateral wall of the sinus. The internal carotid artery lies in the sinus lateral to the dorsum sella, its siphon fitting under the 'shoulder' of the dorsum. The fossa is an indentation in the roof of the sphenoidal sinus, which may be invaded by downward growth of a pituitary tumour.

35. B C D E

Craniopharyngioma is usually calcified and lies above the fossa, hence its old name, 'suprasellar cyst'. It commonly causes optic atrophy by compressing the chiasma or optic nerves, and the consequences of damage to the adjacent hypothalamus include disturbances of appetite, sleep and temperature regulation as well as diabetes insipidus and hyperprolactinaemia. It is important to distinguish craniopharyngioma from other tumours in the area, which (particularly in children) are often highly malignant (e.g., glioma of the optic nerve). Survival after surgical removal and/or irradiation of a craniopharyngioma is often prolonged.

36. A C D E

Hyperprolactinaemia may occur in acromegaly either because the pituitary tumour contains both somatotrophs and lactotrophs or because the tumour interferes with the transport of dopamine (which normally tonically inhibits prolactin release) from the hypothalamus. Dopaminergic agonists such as bromocriptine and pergolide inhibit prolactin release and their long-term use may shrink many prolactinomas. Metoclopramide and other dopaminergic blockers stimulate prolactin release. Hypothalamic damage following external beam radiotherapy frequently leads to hyperprolactinaemia; this is not seen after interstitial irradiation by radioactive yttrium seeds implanted within the gland, as the radiation damage is much more localised.

37. Growth hormone (GH) secretion is normally stimulated by

A somatostatin
B glucagon
C sleep
D glucose
E amino acids

Your answers: A.........B.........C.........D.........E.........

38. In hypopituitarism

A selective gonadotrophin deficiency may be present
B concomitant diabetes insipidus (DI) may be masked by anterior pituitary failure
C adrenal steroid replacement must be started before thyroid replacement
D mineralocorticoid replacement is usually necessary
E in men, androgen replacement will cause masculinisation and restore fertility

Your answers: A.........B.........C.........D.........E.........

39. In active acromegaly

A treatment is not necessary for a small intrasellar tumour which is not expanding
B external beam radiotherapy will normalise growth hormone (GH) levels in most cases within 6 months
C transphenoidal surgical removal is the treatment of choice for large tumours causing visual field constriction
D bromocriptine will normalise (GH) levels in over 90% of cases
E somatostatin analogues can achieve clinical and biochemical remission

Your answers: A.........B.........C.........D.........E.........

Answers overleaf

37. B C E

GH release is normally pulsatile, with increased frequency and amplitude of GH 'spikes' during sleep, exercise and stress. Somatostatin is a physiological inhibitor of GH secretion; its analogues can be used to treat acromegaly. Glucagon stimulates GH secretion, and can be used to test GH reserve in cases where the insulin tolerance test might be hazardous (e.g. ischaemic heart disease). Glucose normally inhibits GH release; failure of GH levels to fall after an oral glucose load is one of the diagnostic criteria of acromegaly, while hypoglycaemia is used as a provocation test of GH reserve. Several amino acids (especially arginine and lysine) stimulate GH secretion.

38. A B C

Isolated deficiencies of gonadotrophins or growth hormone are well described and may be due to failure of secretion of their respective hypothalamic releasing hormones. Concomitant cortisol deficiency reduces the severity of and may even conceal diabetes insipidus, possibly because it lowers glomerular filtration rate. DI may therefore be revealed by adrenal replacement therapy. In combined adrenal and thyroid failure, an adrenal crisis may be precipitated by starting thyroxine replacement therapy before corticosteroids. Aldosterone synthesis and secretion occur in the zona glomerulosa of the adrenal cortex and are largely ACTH-independent. Mineralocorticoid deficiency sufficient to require replacement therapy is therefore rare in hypopituitarism. Fertility depends on the gonadotrophins, which must be replaced for fertility to be achieved.

39. E

Active acromegaly doubles mortality at all ages (due to associated hypertension, diabetes and atheroma) and should therefore be treated in all but the elderly or very frail. GH levels fall relatively slowly after external beam radiotherapy and are normalised in only 40% of cases at 2 years after treatment; interim medical treatment may be necessary. Large extrasellar tumours, especially those compressing the optic chiasma, should be treated surgically; the transfrontal route must be used to allow adequate access. Bromocriptine normalises GH in only about 30% of cases. Long-acting somatostatin analogues can suppress GH levels and cause resolution of acromegaly, and may be effective in some cases unresponsive to bromocriptine.

40. Features of acromegaly include

    A reduced insulin-like growth factor 1 (IGF-1) levels

    B hypercalciuria

    C intestinal polyps

    D multiple skin tags

    E increased libido

    Your answers: A.........B.........C.........D.........E.........

41. Antidiuretic hormone (ADH)

    A is synthesised in the posterior pituitary

    B is a cyclic octapeptide

    C circulates in the blood stream bound to neurophysin

    D is released by carbamazepine

    E is released by ethanol

    Your answers: A.........B.........C.........D.........E.........

42. Nephrogenic diabetes insipidus (NDI)

    A is characterised by low circulating concentrations of antidiuretic hormone (ADH)

    B most commonly shows autosomal dominant inheritance

    C responds to chlorpropamide treatment

    D is aggravated by thiazide diuretics

    E may be caused by lithium treatment

    Your answers: A.........B.........C.........D.........E.........

Answers overleaf

40. B C D

Insulin-like growth factors (the most important is IGF-1) are produced in the liver under the influence of growth hormone (GH) and mediate most of the growth-promoting effects of the hormone. IGF-1 levels are increased in acromegaly but do not always reflect disease severity. Hypercalciuria occurs as a direct renal tubular action of GH; moderate or severe hypercalcaemia suggests hyperparathyroidism associated with the multiple endocrine neoplasia (MEN) 1 syndrome. Intestinal polyps (both benign and malignant) are common in acromegalic patients and should be remembered as possible causes of bowel symptoms and anaemia. Libido is commonly reduced in acromegaly due to impaired gonadotrophin secretion and/or associated hyperprolactinaemia.

41. B D

ADH is synthesised in neurones in the hypothalamus (mostly the supraoptic and paraventricular nuclei). It is transported (bound to neurophysin carrier proteins) along axons descending the pituitary stalk to the posterior pituitary, where it is released into the circulation. Its release is stimulated by high plasma osmolality, hypovolaemia, and by many drugs including morphine, clofibrate and carbamazepine (the last two are used to treat partial cranial diabetes insipidus). ADH secretion is suppressed by naloxone, phenytoin and ethanol.

42. E

NDI is caused by insensitivity to ADH of its target tissues (the distal tubule and collecting ducts). ADH secretion is not defective and levels are generally high-normal or supranormal depending on hydration. NDI has several causes, including inheritance of an X-linked recessive gene, treatment with lithium and demeclocycline (reversible after drug withdrawal) hypercalcaemia and prolonged potassium depletion. Apparently paradoxically, some patients with cranial or nephrogenic DI respond to thiazide diuretics, whose mechanism of action is unknown. Chlorpropamide sensitises the renal tubules to ADH and is used to treat mild cases of cranial DI, but is ineffective in NDI.

43. Short stature in childhood
A is most commonly due to hypopituitarism
B may be due solely to emotional deprivation
C should be treated with growth hormone (GH) if the child's height is below the third centile
D may be due to congenital adrenal hyperplasia
E may be due to hypothyroidism

Your answers: A.........B.........C.........D.........E.........

44. In anorexia nervosa
A loss of pubic hair occurs
B patients may present with primary amenorrhoea
C luteinizing hormone (LH) levels are elevated
D the erythrocyte sedimentation rate (ESR) is high
E cortisol levels are low

Your answers: A.........B.........C.........D.........E.........

45. The following statements are true of Turner's syndrome:
A routine karyotyping may show 46,XX, although the commonest karyotype is 45,XO
B gonadotrophin levels are low
C webbing of the neck is always present
D lymphoedema of hands and feet occurs in the neonate
E 'streak' gonads are present

Your answers: A.........B.........C.........D.........E.........

Answers overleaf

43. B D E

The commonest cause of short stature in childhood physiological slow growth with a delayed pubertal grow spurt, in the absence of any identifiable disease. GH replace ment treatment is indicated only for children persistently belo the third centile for height with a flat GH response during a insulin tolerance test and unfused epiphyses. Rare but trea able causes include emotional deprivation, hypothyroidis and the virilising forms of congenital adrenal hyperplasia (which androgen excess initially accelerates but later term nates growth because of premature epiphyseal fusion).

44. B

Endocrine abnormalities in anorexia nervosa may be due t malnutrition or weight loss. Gonadotrophin levels are low, wit loss of the normal pulsatile pattern of secretion (a profi typical of prepubertal girls). Cortisol levels are high-normal o supranormal (possibly related to depression), and high grow hormone levels may reflect reduced negative feedback on th pituitary by low circulating levels of insulin-like growth factor The eating disorder and weight loss may begin befor menarche and so prevent pubertal gonadotrophin release an the appearance of puberty itself. An elevated ESR sugges organic disease (the ESR is normal or low in anorexia). Loss pubic hair suggests hypopituitarism (in anorexia, pubic hair conserved and fine, dark lanugo hair may appear on the boc and face).

45. A D E

The commonest karyotype in patients with Turner's syndrom is 45,XO, but mosaics such as 45,XO/46,XX have bee described; in these cases, routine karyotyping may mis 45,XO cells if these are in the minority. Turner's syndrom may also occur with 46,XY or 46,XX karyotypes if the chromosome or one of the X chromosomes is structurall defective. Primordial germ cells carrying a Turner karyotyp are not viable and are unable to transform the indiffere gonad into an ovary; the characteristic 'streak' gonads (whic lie behind the broad ligament, in the usual position of th ovary) consist of fibrous tissue and are devoid of germ cell Absent ovarian oestrogen secretion results in sexua immaturity and elevated gonadotrophin levels. The physic signs of Turner's syndrome are variable and include webbin of the neck, cubitus valgus, widely-spaced nipples, variou cardiovascular abnormalities and (in the neonate lymphoedema of the extremities and cystic hygroma.

46. The following statements are true:

A levels of sex-hormone binding globulin are increased in Klinefelter's syndrome

B hypogonadotrophic hypogonadism may be associated with anosmia

C there is a high risk of seminoma in the testicular feminisation syndrome

D azoospermia is invariable in Klinefelter's syndrome

E human chorionic gonadotrophin stimulates testosterone secretion

Your answers: A.........B.........C.........D.........E.........

47. In Graves' disease

A the eye signs usually improve when hyperthyroidism is controlled by antithyroid drugs

B levels of thyroid-stimulating hormone (TSH) are normal

C neonatal hyperthyroidism may result from transplacental passage of maternal thyroxine

D the thyroid is stimulated by antimicrosomal antibodies

E amenorrhoea may occur

Your answers: A.........B.........C.........D.........E.........

48. Features of primary autoimmune hypothyroidism include

A increased incidence of type 1 diabetes and Addison's disease

B pretibial myxoedema

C pericardial effusion

D ataxia

E paranoia and delusions

Your answers: A.........B.........C.........D.........E.........

Answers overleaf

46. A B C E

Circulating testosterone is mainly bound to sex-hormone binding globulin, whose levels are generally inversely related to prevailing testosterone concentrations. Hypogonadotrophic hypogonadism may be associated with impaired or absent sense of smell (Kallman's syndrome). In the testicular feminisation syndrome, the gonads are undescended testes (intra-abdominal or in the inguinal canal) and are therefore at increased risk of malignancy. Typical 47,XXY individuals with Klinefelter's syndrome often show complete seminiferous tubule dysgenesis and therefore azoospermia, but others (especially mosaics) may be relatively well masculinised and rare cases have produced spermatozoa. Human chorionic gonadotrophin (HCG) has LH-like activity and is used to stimulate testosterone secretion by the Leydig cells of the testis.

47. E

In Graves' disease, thyroid stimulation is due to activation of the TSH receptors by autoantibodies which develop against the receptor. By contrast, autoantibodies directed against other thyroid components (e.g. microsomes of the follicular cells or thyroglobulin) cause damage rather than stimulation of the gland. Elevated thyroxine and tri-iodothyronine levels act through negative feedback on the hypothalamus and pituitary to reduce secretion of TSH, whose circulating levels are suppressed to below the normal range (distinguishable by highly sensitive TSH assays). Neonatal hyperthyroidism results from IgG TSH-receptor-stimulating antibodies which cross the placenta and stimulate the fetal thyroid; it resolves spontaneously after some weeks when the antibodies are cleared from the circulation.

48. A C D E

Autoimmune thyroid failure is associated with other organ-specific autoimmune disease; the combination with Addison's disease is referred to as 'Schmidt's syndrome'. Pericardial and pleural effusions and ascites, reversible with thyroid replacement, may occur. Rare neurological complications include bilateral cerebellar damage and 'myxoedema madness' (first described by Richard Asher), which includes hallucinations, agitation, delusions and paranoia. Localised 'myxoedema' consisting of cutaneous hyaluronic acid deposits and most often appearing on the shins, is a feature of Graves' disease.

49. De Quervain's (subacute) thyroiditis is commonly associated with

A elevated ESR

B painless goitre

C dense fibrosis involving the thyroid and adjacent structures

D hyperthyroidism

E increased thyroid uptake of ^{99m}-technetium

Your answers: A.........B.........C.........D.........E.........

50. In the treatment of Cushing's disease (CD)

A long-term metyrapone may be used

B op'-DDD is indicated in patients unfit for surgery

C after bilateral adrenalectomy, Nelson's syndrome is prevented by adequate glucocorticoid replacement

D recurrence of CD after transphenoidal surgery is virtually zero

E yttrium implantation is indicated in the treatment of pituitary tumours compressing the optic chiasma

Your answers: A.........B.........C.........D.........E.........

51. The following statements are true:

A an elevated TSH level excludes the diagnosis of hyperthyroidism

B free thyroxine levels are elevated in normal pregnancy

C most circulating thyroxine is bound to thyroglobulin

D phenytoin treatment may reduce total thyroxine levels

E amiodarone treatment may cause hyperthyroidism

Your answers: A.........B.........C.........D.........E.........

Answers overleaf

49. A D

De Quervain's thyroiditis is caused by viral infections especially mumps, coxsackie and adenoviruses. Most cases present with acute painful enlargement of the thyroid although a rare variant with painless goitre has recently been described. Systemic symptoms (fever, malaise) and an elevated ESR are common. Inflammation of the gland impairs uptake of iodide or technetate but, paradoxically, can cause transient hyperthyroidism due to escape of thyroid hormones. Most cases recover spontaneously but may need non-steroidal anti-inflammatory drugs and sometimes high-dose steroids for local and systemic symptoms. Dense fibrotic infiltration of the thyroid, often involving the trachea and great vessels of the neck, is a feature of Riedel's thyroiditis.

50. A

Metyrapone may be used in the long-term treatment of CD in patients unfit for surgery. Op'-DDD, however, is a toxic adrenolytic drug used only in Cushing's *syndrome* due to adrenal carcinoma. Nelson's syndrome may develop and progress despite high-dose glucocorticoids, but may be treated and possibly prevented by pituitary irradiation. Due to tumour remnant regrowth or missed microadenomata, the recurrence rate for CD after transphenoidal surgery is about 10%. Transfrontal surgery is first-line treatment for tumours with large extrasellar extensions (compression of the chiasm implies a suprasellar extension of at least 10 mm). Interstitial pituitary irradiation using yttrium or gold is effective for intrasellar tumours and those with small ($\leqslant 5$ mm) suprasellar extension.

51. D E

Hyperthyroidism is rarely due to TSH hypersecretion, either from a pituitary adenoma ('TSHoma') or because the pituitary thyrotrophs are insensitive to negative feedback by thyroid hormones. Over 99.9% of circulating T4 is bound to proteins, mainly thyroxine-binding globulin (TBG), prealbumin and albumin. Pregnancy stimulates synthesis of TBG and so increases thyroxine-binding capacity and circulating T4 levels (both bound and total); levels of biologically active free T4 remain normal. Phenytoin binds to TBG and reduces bound and total T4; phenytoin may also reduce free T4, apparently by increasing T4 metabolism. Amiodarone affects thyroid function, through its high iodine content and inhibition of the deiodination of thyroxine (T4) to tri-iodothyronine (T3); either hyper- or hypothyroidism may result.

2. Actions of somatostatin include

A inhibition of growth hormone secretion
B stimulation of insulin secretion
C stimulation of glucagon secretion
D reduced intestinal absorption of nutrients
E direct reduction of thyroxine secretion from the thyroid

Your answers: A.........B.........C.........D.........E.........

3. Common features of Cushing's syndrome due to adrenal carcinoma include

A retarded growth in children
B clitoromegaly
C subconjunctival oedema
D marked hyperpigmentation
E supraclavicular fat pads

Your answers: A.........B.........C.........D.........E.........

4. The following statements are true:

A carbimazole is teratogenic and must be avoided in pregnancy
B skin rashes due to carbimazole are unlikely to recur if therapy is changed to propylthiouracil
C relapse is very rare when carbimazole treatment is continued for two years
D carbimazole is secreted in milk
E symptomatic hypocalcaemia following subtotal thyroidectomy is generally transient

Your answers: A.........B.........C.........D.........E.........

Answers overleaf

52. A D

Somatostatin, a 14 amino acid peptide, was originally isolated from the hypothalamus and named for its ability to inhibit growth hormone (its alternative name is 'somatotrophin release inhibitory factor', or SRIF). It has since been found to inhibit the secretion of a wide range of gut-associated peptides including insulin, glucagon and gastrin and also reduces tumoural secretion of VIP and 5-HT. It reduces TSH secretion, but has no direct effect on the thyroid. Its many effects on the gut include disordered motility and impaired absorption. Steatorrhoea has been reported in acromegalic patients treated long-term with somatostatin analogues.

53. A B C E

Features of cortisol excess in Cushing's syndrome due to all causes include central fat deposition (including the round 'moon' face, 'buffalo' hump and supraclavicular fat pads), subconjunctival oedema (a useful physical sign) and growth retardation or arrest in children. Functional adrenal tumours (both benign adenoma and carcinoma) often produce excess androgen and/or oestrogens in addition to cortisol; marked masculinisation (including clitoromegaly) or feminisation therefore suggests an adrenal tumour rather than pituitary-driven Cushing's disease, in which excess sex steroid production is rare. Primary adrenal over- production of cortisol suppresses ACTH secretion; very high ACTH levels and pronounced hyperpigmentation suggest that Cushing's syndrome is driven by an 'ectopic' source of ACTH such as a lung or pancreatic carcinoma.

54. B D E

There is no evidence that carbimazole is teratogenic, although its dose in pregnancy should be kept as low as possible to avoid fetal hypothyroidism and goitre. As carbimazole is secreted in milk, breast feeding is contraindicated during treatment. Carbimazole frequently causes rashes which mostly resolve when the patient is transferred to propylthiouracil. The relapse rate after a twelve to twenty-four month course of carbimazole is about 50%; relapses may be treated with surgery, a further course of carbimazole, or (in those aged over 40 years) radioiodine. Most cases of hypocalcaemia complicating thyroid surgery are due to temporary parathyroid damage and resolve spontaneously; permanent hypoparathyroidism occurs in less than 1% of cases.

55. The following features suggest inadequate glucocorticoid replacement in Addison's disease:

A insomnia
B tiredness
C loss of appetite
D hypokalaemia
E total daily hydrocortisone dosage of 10 mg

Your answers: A.........B.........C.........D.........E.........

56. Causes of hypokalaemia with increased plasma renin activity include

A psychogenic vomiting
B laxative abuse
C Conn's syndrome
D diuretic abuse
E carbenoxolone treatment

Your answers: A.........B.........C.........D.........E.........

57. In congenital adrenal hyperplasia (CAH)

A 21-hydroxylase deficiency is the commonest variety
B virilisation may be prevented by glucocorticoid treatment
C adrenal crisis may occur within a few days of birth
D blood 17-hydroxyprogesterone concentrations are greatly increased
E severe hypoglycaemia may occur

Your answers: A.........B.........C.........D.........E.........

55. B C

Individual requirements for glucocorticoid replacement var
widely: some patients require as little as 5 mg/day of hydroco
tisone whereas others may need 30 mg/day. Symptom
suggestive of inadequate replacement include tiredness, los
of energy, anorexia, vomiting, headache and 'flu-like' malais
postural hypotension, hyperkalaemia and an elevated bloo
urea concentration may also be present. Insomnia may be du
to over-replacement or to taking the evening dose too lat
Other features of overdosage include excessive weight gai
(especially if with oedema or cushingoid features), hyperter
sion and hypokalaemia.

56. A B D

All the above factors cause hypokalaemia and total bod
potassium depletion which may be profound and symptoma
tic. The important differential diagnosis is from Conn'
syndrome, in which primary adrenal overproduction
aldosterone increases sodium-potassium exchange in th
distal tubule, causing sodium retention (leading to hyperter
sion) and excessive urinary potassium losses. In primar
hyperaldosteronism, plasma renin activity is suppressed b
sodium and water overload, as is also the case with carbeno>
olone, a steroidal compound with similar sodium-retaining an
potassium-losing effects. Carbenoxolone causes hyperter
sion and hypokalaemia similar to Conn's syndrome, b
plasma aldosterone levels are suppressed. In conditions A,
and D, sodium and water losses and the resulting intravascu
lar volume depletion stimulate plasma renin activity.

57. A B C D E

CAH is a group of diseases due to inherited deficiencies
various steroid biosynthetic enzymes, of which 21-hydro>
ylase is the most commonly affected. The manifestations
CAH depend on the site of the enzyme defect and on th
relative effects of 'upstream' precursor excesses and of en
product deficiency. Cortisol deficiency may be severe an
fatal in the neonatal period. With 21-hydroxylase defect
17-hydroxyprogesterone and other androgens accumulat
causing virilisation. Glucocorticoid treatment not only replace
cortisol but also suppresses androgenic precursors, and ca
prevent virilism; 17-hydroxyprogesterone and testosteror
levels are useful guides to adjusting dosage. Life-threatenir
hypoglycaemia may accompany cortisol deficiency due
intercurrent illness or omission of steroids.

58. In primary hyperparathyroidism

A osteitis fibrosa cystica occurs in most cases

B multiple small lytic skull lesions are common in severe disease

C peptic ulceration may occur

D serum alkaline phosphatase activity is increased in most asymptomatic cases

E surgery is the treatment of choice if serum calcium exceeds 3.0 mmol/l

Your answers: A.........B.........C.........D.........E.........

59. Idiopathic hypoparathyroidism is associated with

A increased incidence of Addison's disease

B chronic mucocutaneous candidiasis

C basal ganglia calcification, commonly causing Parkinsonism

D short fourth and fifth metacarpals

E good response of hypocalcaemia to calcium and vitamin D treatment

Your answers: A.........B.........C.........D.........E.........

60. In the treatment of hypercalcaemia

A mithramycin is useful long-term therapy

B calcitonin may be useful acutely

C high-dose prednisolone (60 mg/day) will reduce serum calcium acutely in primary hyperparathyroidism

D severe hypocalcaemia may follow removal of a single parathyroid adenoma

E peritoneal dialysis is effective

Your answers: A.........B.........C.........D.........E.........

Answers overleaf

58. B C E

Severe bone disease in primary hyperparathyroidism is relatively rare: osteitis fibrosa cystica occurs in under 10% of cases. The skull commonly shows thinning of the calvarium, subperiosteal erosions and multiple small lucencies (the 'pepperpot skull'). Peptic ulceration may result from hypercalcaemia itself or from an associated gastrinoma (Zollinger-Ellison syndrome). Serum alkaline phosphatase is increased only with significant bone disease and is normal in most asymptomatic cases. Surgery is indicated when serum calcium exceeds 3.0 mmol/l because of bone and renal disease and because medical treatment (low calcium diet, frusemide, sodium cellulose phosphate) is generally ineffective.

59. A B E

Hypoparathyroidism due to polyglandular autoimmune disease is associated with hypothyroidism, Addison's disease, type 1 diabetes, primary ovarian failure and pernicious anaemia. Chronic mucocutaneous candidiasis is common in autoimmune hypoparathyroidism and in di George's syndrome. Calcification of the basal ganglia occurs in both hypoparathyroidism and pseudohypoparathyroidism (which is due to target organ resistance to parathyroid hormone, not to parathyroid failure), but Parkinsonism is rare. Several somatic features (including short stature, 'moon-face' and short metacarpals and metatarsals) occur in pseudohypoparathyroidism, but not in true hypoparathyroidism. Both hypoparathyroidism and pseudohypoparathyroidism are treated with calcium and vitamin D derivatives, eg. alfacalcidol.

60. B D E

Serum calcium concentrations may be reduced acutely by calcitonin, mithramycin and peritoneal or haemodialysis. However, neither drug is suitable for long-term use: patients soon become refractory to calcitonin, and mithramycin is toxic to liver, kidney and platelets. High-dose steroids are effective in hypercalcaemia due to malignancy, myeloma, and sarcoidosis, but not in hyperparathyroidism. Profound hypocalcaemia, hypomagnesaemia and hypophosphataemia, often lasting several days, may follow surgical removal of overactive parathyroid glands especially in patients with extensive bone disease. This 'hungry bones' syndrome is due to rapid remineralisation of the decalcified skeleton, and intense osteoblastic activity causes a characteristic rise in alkaline phosphatase.

61. The following statements are true of Paget's disease:
A patients may become refractory to calcitonin treatment
B deafness may occur
C cardiac failure is a complication
D hypercalcaemia is common
E serum alkaline phosphate may be normal in active disease

Your answers: A.........B.........C.........D.........E.........

62. Features of the multiple endocrine neoplasia (MEN) syndrome type 1 include
A parathyroid hyperplasia
B multiple neuromata around the eyes and mouth
C acromegaly
D medullary carcinoma of the thyroid
E profuse watery diarrhoea

Your answers: A.........B.........C.........D.........E.........

63. In the differential diagnosis of hypoglycaemia
A high C-peptide concentrations in the presence of hypoglycaemia suggest factitious insulin administration
B a high ratio of proinsulin to insulin in a fasting blood sample is a feature of insulinoma
C nesidioblastosis should be considered in the neonate or infant
D the tolbutamide test is useful in the diagnosis of insulinoma
E a 72-hour fast fails to produce hypoglycaemia in up to 20% of insulinomas

Your answers: A.........B.........C.........D.........E.........

Answers overleaf

61. A B C E

With prolonged use some patients become resistant to calcitonin, sometimes because of anti-calcitonin antibodies. Pagetic bone overgrowth may compress structures passing through bony foramina, such as cranial nerves and the spinal cord. The diversion of blood flow to the highly-vascular pagetic bones may cause 'steal' syndromes and occasionally high-output cardiac failure. Hypercalcaemia is rare unless patients are immobilised or suffer fractures. Alkaline phosphatase activity is within the normal range in nearly 10% of untreated patients, but will generally fall after starting calcitonin treatment and so can still be used to monitor therapy.

62. A C E

The MEN 1 syndrome comprises two or more of the following: parathyroid tumours (hyperplasia is commoner than adenoma, and carcinoma is very rare), pituitary tumours, and pancreatic endocrine tumours. The latter include insulinoma, glucagonoma, gastrinoma, carcinoid, VIPoma (causing the Verner-Morrison syndrome of watery diarrhoea, hypokalaemia and achlorhydria) and rare tumours producing growth hormone releasing hormone, which can cause acromegaly. Medullary carcinoma of the thyroid, phaeochromocytoma and parathyroid tumours define the MEN-2 syndrome multiple facial neuromata (especially of the eyelids, tongue and lips) occur in a variant of MEN-2 syndrome (MEN-2b, or MEN-3).

63. B C

In both normal and neoplastic B-cells, proinsulin is cleaved enzymatically to produce equimolar amounts of insulin and C-peptide. Hypoglycaemia caused by exogenous insulin (which contains virtually no C-peptide) inhibits pancreatic insulin release and circulating C-peptide levels are therefore low. In insulinomas, defective post-translational processing of proinsulin may allow proinsulin to be secreted in addition to insulin and C-peptide. Virtually all patients with an insulinoma will become hypoglycaemic (venous plasma glucose concentration $\leqslant 1.7$ mmol/l) and neuroglycopaenic during a 72-hour fast. The tolbutamide test is dangerous and now obsolete. Nesidioblastosis is diffuse B-cell hyperplasia occurring throughout the pancreas, in contrast to the focal B-cell proliferation of insulinomas. Although rare, it is in early childhood more common than discrete insulinomas.

64. Features of the VIPoma syndrome include
A hypokalaemia
B alkalosis
C hypoglycaemia
D increased gastric acid secretion
E provocation of VIP release by somatostatin

Your answers: A.........B.........C.........D.........E.........

65. Phaeochromocytoma
A is excluded by a normal CT scan of the adrenals
B may secrete dopamine
C is associated with islet-cell tumours
D pending surgery, should be treated by ß-blockade
E may be localised on an IVP

Your answers: A.........B.........C.........D.........E.........

66. The following statements are true:
A calcitonin-gene related peptide has a potent calcium-lowering effect
B diarrhoea is common in the gastrinoma syndrome
C DDAVP is a powerful vasoconstrictor
D thromboembolic disease is common in the glucagonoma syndrome
E high gastrin levels are associated with pernicious anaemia

Your answers: A.........B.........C.........D.........E.........

Answers overleaf

64. A

The VIPoma (Verner-Morrison) syndrome is also known descriptively as 'pancreatic cholera' or the Watery Diarrhoea-Hypokalaemia-Achlorhydria (WDHA) syndrome. Profuse secretory diarrhoea causes massive intestinal loss of water, potassium, sodium and bicarbonate, leading to hypovolaemia, hypokalaemia and total body potassium depletion and acidosis. Reduced or absent gastric acid secretion is a direct effect of VIP. Associated metabolic features include glucose intolerance (VIP causes mild insulin resistance) and hypercalcaemia. Somatostatin suppresses tumoural VIP secretion (like most gut regulatory peptides; somatostatin has been nicknamed 'endocrine cyanide') and its analogues are used to treat the VIPoma syndrome.

65. B E

Ten per cent of phaeochromocytomas lie outside the adrenal medulla, and even those in the classical site may not be detected by CT scan. The presence of large tumours may be deduced from displacement of the renal outline on an IVP. In addition to adrenaline (which predominates in adrenal phaeochromocytomas) and noradrenaline (extra-adrenal tumours), dopamine may be secreted, especially by malignant tumours. Phaeochromocytomas occur in association with medullary carcinoma of the thyroid and parathyroid tumours (=MEN-2), but not with pancreatic endocrine or pituitary tumours (=MEN-1). Treatment with ß-blockers alone is hazardous: removal of ß-adrenergic vasodilation in skeletal muscle may cause a hypertensive crisis. Treatment should therefore start with an α-blocker (e.g. phenoxybenzamine), to which a ß-blocker may be added to control tachycardia.

66. B D E

Calcitonin-gene related peptide is a peptide encoded within the calcitonin gene complex, but with entirely different actions. It has no effect on calcium metabolism but is a powerful vasodilator. Secretory diarrhoea occurs in most patients with gastrinoma and is mainly due to acid hypersecretion. DDAVP is an analogue of arginine vasopressin which, unlike the native peptide has virtually no vasoconstrictor activity and can therefore be used in patients with ischaemic heart disease. Gastrin release is inhibited by the presence of acid in the stomach; reduced acid secretion (as in the atrophic gastritis of pernicious anaemia) therefore stimulates gastrin secretion.

RENAL MEDICINE

Indicate your answers by putting T (True), F (False) or D (Don't know) in the spaces provided.

67. Recognised causes of acute renal failure include
- A regular ingestion of paracetamol for a prolonged period
- B thiazide diuretics
- C minimal change glomerulonephritis
- D antifreeze poisoning
- E psoriasis

Your answers: A.........B.........C.........D.........E.........

68. Frusemide
- A increases sodium excretion by direct inhibition of the sodium pump in the loop of Henlé
- B decreases free water clearance in the nephron
- C reduces the passive reabsorption of water from distal tubule and collecting duct
- D decreases renal calcium reabsorption
- E is a potassium 'sparing' diuretic

Your answers: A.........B.........C.........D.........E.........

69. Characteristics of the hepatorenal syndrome include
- A intratubular deposition of bilirubin
- B oliguria
- C daily urinary sodium losses exceeding 50 mmol
- D good prognosis following renal transplantation
- E diuresis following albumin infusion

Your answers: A.........B.........C.........D.........E.........

Answers overleaf

67. A B C D E

Paracetamol alone has been described as a cause of analgesic nephropathy which may present as acute renal failure owing to bilateral ureteric obstruction by sloughed papillae. Thiazide diuretics, frusemide, the non-steroidal anti-inflammatory drugs, phenindione, sulphonamides and the penicillins, especially methicillin are the drugs most commonly associated with acute allergic interstitial nephritis. Acute renal failure in minimal change glomerulonephritis seems to result from tubular obstruction owing to interstitial oedema. Poisoning with ethylene glycol or methanol causes renal oxalosis. Severe psoriasis, like other skin diseases, can cause urate nephropathy.

68. B C D

Frusemide acts primarily on the co-transport pathway for Na/K/Cl co-transport in the ascending limb of the loop of Henlé. As a consequence of the reduced sodium reabsorption the concentrating ability of the kidney is diminished leading to a fall in water reabsorption from the distal tubule and collecting duct. The ascending limb is the site of formation of free water since sodium is reabsorbed without water. By inhibiting sodium reabsorption frusemide reduces free water formation. Sodium reabsorption is inhibited proximal to the potassium secreting site (distal tubule) and the increase in tubular sodium will stimulate potassium loss. Frusemide also inhibits calcium reabsorption in the loop.

69. B

The hepatorenal syndrome results from reduced cortical perfusion secondary to the accumulation of a vasoactive substance, thought to be endotoxin, which is normally cleared in the liver. Oliguria and a daily urine sodium excretion of under 10 mmol are the rule. The syndrome only resolves if there is a dramatic improvement in hepatic function and so liver transplantation is the treatment of choice. Interestingly, the kidneys of a patient with hepatorenal syndrome will function if transplanted into a recipient with a normal liver. Although the blood volume is frequently low, plasma expanders rarely improve renal function.

0. In the proximal tubule

A the filtrate becomes increasingly hypertonic

B the brush border has a low density of active sodium pumping sites

C acetazolamide is maximally effective

D glucose reabsorption always parallels the filtered glucose load

E bicarbonate ions are passively transported across the brush border

Your answers: A.........B.........C.........D.........E.........

1. The following are typical features of the haemolytic uraemic syndrome:

A reticulocytosis

B low serum haptoglobin

C thrombocytosis

D fragmentation of red cells

E positive Coombs' test

Your answers: A.........B.........C.........D.........E.........

72. In patients with end-stage renal failure treated by haemodialysis

A red-cell lifespan is reduced

B over 10% develop entrapment neuropathy

C cardiac output is characteristically decreased

D the serum gastrin concentration is low

E the incidence of adenocarcinoma of the kidney is increased

Your answers: A.........B.........C.........D.........E.........

Answers overleaf

70. B C

Sodium and water reabsorption occur isotonically across th
cells of the proximal tubule and the filtrate is thus isoton
throughout. Active sodium transport occurs in the basolater
membrane, not the brush border. Glucose reabsorptic
parallels the filtered glucose load, until all carrier sites a
occupied (and T_m is reached) after which glucose appears
the urine. Acetazolamide is a proximally acting diuretic whic
reduces bicarbonate reabsorption by inhibition of carbon
anhydrase. The brush border is impermeable to HCO_3^- ion
which gain entry to the cell by combining with H^+ to form H_2
and CO_2. These diffuse freely across the brush border.

71. A B D

In haemolytic uraemic syndrome there is evidence
intravascular haemolysis owing to microangiopathy with frag
mentation of red cells, a low serum haptoglobin concentratio
and a marginally raised serum indirect bilirubin concentration
Patients with this syndrome differ from those with othe
causes of renal failure in their ability to mount a reticulocyt
response. The platelet count is reduced by consumption
microthrombi. There is no association with autoimmun
haemolytic anaemia.

72. A B E

The causes of anaemia in renal failure include relativ
erythropoietin deficiency, retention of inhibitors of erythr
poiesis, deficiency of haematinics, excessive blood loss ar
haemolysis. Entrapment neuropathy, particularly carpal tur
nel syndrome, occurs in about 15% of chronical
haemodialysed patients; the cause in many cases
amyloidosis owing to ß2-microglobulin deposition. The ca
diac output is increased in response to anaemia; it may b
higher still in patients whose arterio-venous fistulae have larg
flows. Gastrin, like other peptide hormones, is metabolised
the kidney and hypergastrinaemia is one factor predisposin
to peptic ulceration in uraemic subjects. Multiple renal cys
develop in about 40% of patients who have been dialysed f
over 10 years; neoplasms occur within cysts in 30% and 10
of these are malignant.

3. Filtration at the glomerulus

A results from a net filtration pressure of 10 mm Hg in normal subjects

B is favoured if a molecule is positively charged

C results in a filtration fraction of 40% in normal subjects

D results in the formation of approximately 360 litres of filtrate per day in normal man

E is reduced by efferent arteriolar constriction

Your answers: A.........B.........C.........D.........E.........

4. Patients with aluminium intoxication have

A macrocytic anaemia

B always been haemodialysed

C osteomalacia responsive to 1,25-dihydroxycholecalciferol

D myoclonic spasms

E predominant sensory symptoms

Your answers: A.........B.........C.........D.........E.........

5. Indications for urgent dialysis in uraemic patients include

A asterixis

B itching

C pericarditis

D peripheral neuropathy

E hiccoughing

Your answers: A.........B.........C.........D.........E.........

Answers overleaf

73. A B

The pressure favouring filtration at the glomerulus = hydrostatic pressure − (oncotic pressure + Bowman's capsule pressure) = 45-(25+10) = 10 mm Hg. The basement membrane consists of negatively charged glycoproteins (including sialic acid) and collagen. The filtration fraction = GFR/renal plasma flow = 125/600 or 20% in normal man. Daily filtration is approximately 180 litres. Efferent arteriolar constriction increases the GFR and may be involved in the phenomenon of 'autoregulation' if renal perfusion pressure falls.

74. D

The aluminium intoxication syndrome is most common in patients haemodialysed in areas where aluminium salts have been added to the local water supply as flocculating agents. Aluminium-containing phosphate binders have also been implicated in the aetiopathogenesis, and it has been described in patients managed conservatively or by peritoneal dialysis. It may cause a hypochromic microcytic anaemia by interfering with haem synthesis, bone disease characterised by osteomalacia, multiple fractures and vitamin D resistance and dialysis dementia which usually presents with dysarthria, ataxia, myoclonus and fits.

75. A C E

Asterixis and hiccoughing are signs of uraemic encephalopathy and so are indications for dialysis. Pericarditis is also life-threatening as cardiac tamponade may occur owing to bleeding from the inflamed pericardium. This may be exacerbated by anticoagulants used during haemodialysis and so reduced heparinisation, regional heparinisation of the extracorporeal circulation or peritoneal dialysis should be used. Itching is usually a manifestation of secondary hyperparathyroidism and may be worsened acutely during haemodialysis. Peripheral neuropathy seldom resolves even with intensive dialysis and is an indication for urgent renal transplantation.

6. Antidiuretic hormone (ADH)

A is produced in response to dehydration of osmoreceptors in the hypothalamus

B production is increased by nicotine

C is more effective in concentrating the urine in cases of adrenal insufficiency

D is normally present at a concentration of 6-8 pg/ml

E increases the reabsorption of solute free water

Your answers: A.........B.........C.........D.........E.........

7. In patients with renal failure the following statements are correct:

A nitrofurantoin is a suitable antibiotic for the treatment of urinary tract infection

B hyperuricaemia requires treatment with allopurinol

C 1,25-dihydroxycholecalciferol increases intestinal absorption of phosphate

D folic acid supplements are required

E frusemide increases glomerular filtration rate

Your answers: A.........B.........C.........D.........E.........

8. The pathway for the transport of organic acids in the nephron

A depends on the formation of secretory vesicles

B is an example of carrier mediated transport

C may be useful in the assessment of the glomerular filtration rate

D is the principal pathway for the excretion of acetazolamide

E is present only in the distal tubule

Your answers: A.........B.........C.........D.........E.........

Answers overleaf

76. A B E

ADH is produced in response to serum hyperosmolarity and subsequent dehydration of osmoreceptors located near the site of formation of ADH in the hypothalamus. Normal plasma ADH is approximately 4 pg/ml and is increased by several pharmacological agents including nicotine, morphine and barbiturates. ADH increases water reabsorption in the collecting duct leading to negative free water clearance, or an increase in solute free water reabsorption. Glucocorticoids enhance collecting duct permeability and in adrenal insufficiency basal permeability is increased and ADH less effective.

77. C

If the glomerular filtration rate is below 30 ml/min, levels of nitrofurantoin in the urine are inadequate and the incidence of side effects becomes unacceptably high. Although hyperuricaemia occurs in most uraemic patients, gout is rare owing to neutrophil dysfunction and so allopurinol is unnecessary. Vitamin D increases intestinal absorption of both calcium and phosphate, and so the serum phosphate should be lowered before vitamin D is given to reduce the risk of ectopic calcification. Although folic acid is a small dialysable molecule, dietary intake generally replaces losses adequately. Frusemide has diuretic, natriuretic and kaliuretic effects in uraemia but does not increase glomerular filtration.

78. B D

The organic acid transport pathway is especially important in clinical medicine as it is the principal pathway for the excretion of many drugs including acetazolamide, frusemide and penicillin. Transport is energy requiring and involves a carrier which transports organic acids from blood to cytoplasm. It is the site of elimination of para-amino hippuric acid which is almost totally extracted from the blood and may thus be used in the determination of renal plasma flow.

Relative contraindications to continuous ambulatory peritoneal dialysis include

A obesity

B rheumatoid arthritis

C previous appendicectomy

D chronic obstructive airways disease

E peripheral vascular disease

Your answers: A.........B.........C.........D.........E.........

The clearance

A of a substance by the kidney is defined as the volume of blood cleared of that substance in one minute

B of a compound which is freely filtered by the kidney and neither secreted nor reabsorbed is a measure of the renal plasma flow

C of inulin is normal when plasma inulin = 0.02 mg/ml, urinary inulin = 2.5 mg/ml, and the urinary flow rate = 60 ml/hr

D of urea is an accurate estimate of the GFR in the hydrated state

E of penicillin is reduced by probenicid

Your answers: A.........B.........C.........D.........E.........

The dose of the following drugs should be modified in uraemic subjects:

A vancomycin

B cimetidine

C bumetanide

D digitoxin

E indomethacin

Your answers: A.........B.........C.........D.........E.........

Answers overleaf

79. A B D E

Each litre of 'isotonic' peritoneal dialysis fluid contains 13.6 of glucose, much of which is absorbed, and so obesity is serious complication especially in previously overweig patients. Patients with severe manual deformities may n have the dexterity required to change dialysis bags witho introducing infection. Previous abdominal surgery is only contraindication if adhesions or a potential infection risk suc as a fistula or stoma are present. The large volume of fluid the peritoneal cavity impairs ventilation by splinting th diaphragms, and exacerbates peripheral vascular insuf ciency.

80. A C E

The definition of clearance is correct. The clearance of substance freely filtered but not secreted or reabsorbed by th kidney (e.g. inulin) is an accurate estimate of GFR. Ren plasma flow is measured from the clearance of a compoun which is filtered and secreted by the kidney (e.g. PAH). Th formula for inulin clearance $= \dfrac{U_{in} \times V}{P_{in}}$ where U_{in} and P_{in} are th concentrations of inulin in urine and plasma and V is the ra of urine flow/min. Clearance thus calculated is 125 ml/min an is a measurement of the normal GFR. Urea is reabsorbed b the kidney even in the hydrated state (approx 40%) and th clearance is much lower than the GFR. Probenicid decrease penicillin secretion and excretion in the distal tubule an therefore decreases its clearance.

81. A B C

Vancomycin accumulates in renal failure and is nephrotox and ototoxic. Cimetidine may precipitate an acu encephalopathy; ranitidine is also retained but toxicity is les Higher doses of loop diuretics such as bumetanide ar needed to effect a diuresis in uraemic patients. Digitoxin cleared in the liver, but 10% is metabolised to digoxin and s although modification of the dose is seldom needed, leve should be monitored. Indomethacin does not accumulate renal failure but it should be used with great caution in view the increased prevalence of peptic ulceration in uraemia.

82. The following will result in an increase in urinary sodium excretion:
   A a decrease in renal sympathetic nervous activity
   B a rise of 15 mm Hg in renal arterial pressure
   C a 10% increase in glomerular filtration rate (GFR)
   D a decrease in the plasma protein concentration
   E an increase in venous volume

   Your answers: A.........B.........C.........D.........E.........

83. When imaging the renal tract of uraemic subjects
   A renal obstruction is best diagnosed by static radionuclide scanning
   B dehydration is indicated to improve the quality of intravenous urograms
   C lateral displacement of the ureters is characteristic of retroperitoneal fibrosis
   D large kidneys exclude a diagnosis of chronic renal failure
   E coarse kidney scarring is diagnostic of reflux nephropathy

   Your answers: A.........B.........C.........D.........E.........

84. IgA mesangial glomerulonephritis
   A is the most common form of glomerulonephritis
   B is complicated by end-stage failure in over 50% of those affected
   C characteristically demonstrates glomerular crescents during episodes of macroscopic haematuria
   D causes loin pain owing to bleeding from peripheral renal arteries
   E has a worse prognosis when proteinuria exceeds 1 g/day

   Your answers: A.........B.........C.........D.........E.........

Answers overleaf

82. **A B D E**

Despite the mechanism of 'autoregulation' which maintains renal blood flow and the GFR within narrow limits, small increases in the renal arterial pressure are paralleled by decreases in proximal sodium reabsorption and sodium excretion is increased. An increase in venous volume stimulates baroreceptors in the atria and in renal capillaries leading to increased sodium excretion by decreased proximal reabsorption and decreased sympathetic tone. Decreased plasma oncotic pressure reduces proximal sodium reabsorption.

83. **None are correct**

The screening test for renal obstruction is ultrasound; if the collecting system is dilated, pressure studies may be needed to confirm the diagnosis. Dehydration may precipitate acute on chronic renal failure owing to contrast nephropathy especially in the elderly, arteriopaths, diabetics and patients with myeloma. The ureters are deviated medially in retroperitoneal fibrosis. Chronically diseased kidneys usually shrink but they characteristically remain large in diabetes, amyloidosis and polycystic kidney disease. Causes of coarse kidney scarring include reflux nephropathy, obstructive uropathy and papillary necrosis.

84. **A C E**

IgA nephropathy appears more common than other forms of glomerulonephritis, at least in Europe, North America and Australasia. Only about 25% progress to end-stage renal failure; poor prognostic factors include uraemia at presentation, heavy proteinuria and frequent episodes of macroscopic haematuria. Acute exacerbations usually coincide with infections or excessive exercise and are characterised histologically by glomerular crescents, and clinically by loin pain owing to swelling of the kidney, macroscopic haematuria and heavy proteinuria. The loin pain-haematuria syndrome which is due to bleeding from microaneurysms of the peripheral renal arteries is a different disease.

85. Rapidly progressive glomerulonephritis

A may be precipitated by exposure to hydrocarbons
B is always associated with antibodies to the glomerular basement membrane
C is associated with haemoptysis most commonly in smokers
D has a worse prognosis if the patient is anuric
E may present with the nephrotic syndrome

Your answers: A.........B.........C.........D.........E.........

86. Membranous glomerulopathy

A is typically accompanied by circulating immune complexes
B is the glomerulopathy most commonly associated with Hodgkin's disease
C remits spontaneously in over 50% of affected adults
D is a recognised cause of hypertension in the absence of renal failure
E is a recognised cause of macroscopic haematuria

Your answers: A.........B.........C.........D.........E.........

87. The response of the kidney to an acid load

A involves an increase in urinary free hydrogen ion secretion until a minimum pH of 3.8 is achieved
B leads to an increase in the chloride-anion gap
C results in the generation of $H_2PO_4^-$ ions in the urine
D leads to increased synthesis of glutamic acid in the cells of the distal tubule
E is hampered by the respiratory response

Your answers: A.........B.........C.........D.........E.........

Answers overleaf

85. A C D E

There is an increased incidence of prior exposure to volatile hydrocarbons in patients developing most forms of glomerulonephritis including rapidly progressive glomerulonephritis. One third of patients have anti-glomerular basement membrane disease, one third have underlying systemic disease such as vasculitis, systemic lupus erythematosis, cryoglobulinaemia or malignancy, and the remainder are cryptogenic. Goodpasture's syndrome is more common in smokers. An acute nephritic or nephrotic onset is usual with progression to end-stage renal failure within six months. Response to treatment is variable but less likely in anuric patients and those with anti-glomerular basement membrane disease.

86. D E

Membranous nephropathy is associated with immune complexes formed in situ between cationic antigens trapped beneath the glomerular epithelium and circulating antibodies. It may complicate malignant disease but minimal change nephropathy and amyloidosis are more commonly associated with lymphomas. Most present with nephrotic syndrome but many also have haematuria (which may be macroscopic), hypertension and uraemia. Spontaneous remission occurs in 67% of children but only 25% of adults.

87. B C D E

Metabolic acidosis increases tubular hydrogen ion secretion until the concentration gradient favouring secretion falls to zero at pH 4.5. In the distal tubule the titration of phosphate ions and ammonia increases i.e. $HPO_4^{2-} + H^+ \rightarrow H_2PO_4^-$ and $NH_3 + H^+ \rightarrow NH_4^+$, thus achieving net hydrogen ion excretion. The ammonia is produced by increased synthesis of glutamic acid from glutamine. The respiratory response of hyperventilation leads to a fall in plasma $[H^+]$ thus reducing H^+ ion secretion in the nephron and blunting the renal response. As a large amount of sodium is excreted in combination with phosphate and ammonia, urinary $[Cl^-]$ will be low and the chloride-anion gap high.

88. Ascent to 10,000 ft can lead to a reduction in arterial pCO_2 in normal people. The response in the kidney

A leads to a fall in plasma $[HCO_3^-]$

B is corrective rather than compensatory

C results in arterial pCO_2 returning to normal

D leads to a fall in plasma pH

E occurs predominantly in the proximal tubules

Your answers: A.........B.........C.........D.........E.........

89. Active tuberculosis of the urinary tract

A is a recognised cause of renal calculi

B may cause ureteric obstruction when treated

C is a contraindication to renal transplantation

D is a recognised cause of urge incontinence

E is associated with a normal chest X-ray in over 50% of cases

Your answers: A.........B.........C.........D.........E.........

90. In cystinuria

A stones are radio-opaque

B acidification of the urine may dissolve stones

C penicillamine increases the excretion of free cysteine

D staghorn calculi indicate associated urinary tract infection

E calcium phosphate stones are a recognised complication

Your answers: A.........B.........C.........D.........E.........

Answers overleaf

88. A D E

The reduction in arterial pCO_2 will lower the plasma HCO_3^- and increase pH (respiratory alkalosis). The increased pH will reduce the rate of renal H^+ secretion, less bicarbonate will be reabsorbed and a further fall in plasma HCO_3^- will occur. This will correct the pH. The overall response is compensatory as arterial pCO_2 remains low and plasma HCO_3^- is much reduced. The main site of bicarbonate reabsorption is proximal.

89. A B C D E

Renal tuberculosis may present clinically or radiologically with calculous disease. Since healing is by fibrosis, lesions within the ureter may form strictures especially during the first six weeks of treatment. Active tuberculosis anywhere contraindicates renal transplantation. Transplant recipients with quiescent disease require continuous prophylaxis; isoniazid is preferred to rifampicin since the latter increases metabolism of cyclosporin A. Tuberculous cystitis may cause disabling frequency and dysuria necessitating urinary diversion or a bladder augmentation. There is no radiological sign of pulmonary tuberculosis in about 60% of cases.

90. A E

Cystine stones are radio-opaque, frequently bilateral and can enlarge to fill the whole pelvi-calyceal system. The staghorn calculi complicating infection with urease producing bacteria are composed of triple phosphate. Treatment includes a high fluid intake, alkalinisation of the urine, and penicillamine. The latter forms a highly soluble disulphide with cysteine. Calcium phosphate stones are a complication of alkalinisation of the urine.

91. Features of primary hyperoxaluria include

A autosomal dominant inheritance
B excessive interstitial absorption of oxalate
C a consistent reduction of urinary oxalate excretion with high doses of pyridoxine
D heart block
E a characteristic abnormal facies

Your answers: A.........B.........C.........D.........E.........

92. The following statements are true:

A the average daily stool weight of a Western adult is 500 g
B total gut secretions are around 7.5 litres daily
C there is no sodium absorption in the colon
D the water absorption capacity of the colon is approximately 1.5 l/day
E potassium concentration is higher in faecal than ileal fluid

Your answers: A.........B.........C.........D.........E.........

93. Recognised associations of distal renal tubular acidosis include

A Sjögren's syndrome
B rickets
C hypercitraturia
D cranial diabetes insipidus
E pseudohypoparathyroidism

Your answers: A.........B.........C.........D.........E.........

91. D

Primary hyperoxaluria is an autosomal recessively inherited condition in which there is increased endogenous production of oxalate. Only some patients are pyridoxine-sensitive. Recurrent calculi lead to renal failure and systemic oxalosis. Death typically results from deposition of oxalate in blood vessels and the conducting tissue of the heart

92. B E

Approximately 9 litres of fluid a day enter the small intestine, 7.5 litres in the diet. Less than 1 litre enters the colon, although the water absorptive capacity of the colon is 3-6 l/day. The colon reabsorbs both water and sodium, but potassium tends to be lost. As a result of colonic activity, daily stool weight on an average Western diet is less than 200 g/day with around 70% water.

93. A B C

Distal renal tubular acidosis may be either congenital or associated with antibodies against tubular basement membrane. This latter form presents usually in adult women and is associated with other autoimmune phenomena including chronic active hepatitis, thyroiditis, fibrosing alveolitis and Sjögren's syndrome. Rickets occurs in the congenital form owing to acidosis or occasionally an associated proximal tubular phosphate leak. Other manifestations of distal tubular dysfunction such as nephrogenic diabetes insipidus may co-exist. A normal urinary citrate virtually excludes the diagnosis.

4. Nephroblastoma

A is more common in adults than children

B causes hypertension in over 50% of cases

C is characteristically sensitive to chemotherapy

D is bilateral in over 20% of cases

E calcifies in over 50% of cases

Your answers: A.........B.........C.........D.........E.........

5. The following statements are true:

A increased sympathetic nervous tone enhances intestinal propulsive activity

B in the fasting state, there is no intestinal motor activity

C a 'migrating motor complex' takes around 15 minutes to traverse the length of the small intestine

D the intrinsic rate of depolarisation of intestinal smooth muscle is similar throughout the intestine

E 'migrating motor complexes' are abolished by food

Your answers: A.........B.........C.........D.........E.........

6. Children with reflux nephropathy are more likely to progress rapidly to end-stage renal failure if

A there are associated posterior urethral valves

B antibiotics are started promptly when infection is documented

C daily urine protein excretion exceeds 1 g

D haematuria is present

E dietary protein intake is low

Your answers: A.........B.........C.........D.........E.........

Answers overleaf

94. B C

Nephroblastoma is a disease of children. Hypertension resul
from high circulating renin; erythrocytosis may also occu
10% are bilateral and unlike renal adenocarcinomas the
seldom calcify. The response to chemotherapy is excelle
with a 5 year survival of about 90%

95. E

Gut motility is vital for normal passage of food through th
intestine. In the fasting state, 'migrating motor complexe
(MMC) occur about every 100 minutes usually starting in th
stomach or duodenum and progressing to the terminal ileu
in 90-120 minutes. This periodic activity is abolished by food
be replaced by irregular localised contractions to aid mixing
food. The intrinsic rate of muscle depolarisation vari
throughout the intestine, the highest rate is set by the duod
nal pacemaker and the rate decreases to the terminal ileun

96. A B C

Reflux nephropathy generally results from intra-renal reflux
infected urine during childhood and is more likely to progress
associated with obstruction. Prophylactic antibiotics should
given continuously to suppress infection. Haematuria has lit
prognostic value but proteinuria suggests the development
focal segmental glomerulosclerosis and hyalinosis whi
heralds inexorable progression to end-stage renal failur
Restriction of dietary protein slows progression of th
glomerular lesion.

7. Children presenting with the nephrotic syndrome

A should not be treated without a prior renal biopsy

B have renal insufficiency if the glomerular filtration rate is normal

C will not respond to cyclophosphamide if non-responsive to steroids

D are unlikely to have minimal change glomerulopathy if they are hypertensive

E have post-streptococcal glomerulonephritis if their antistreptolysin O titre is raised

Your answers: A.........B.........C.........D.........E.........

8. Infantile polycystic kidney disease

A sparing one kidney is recognised

B is the most common cause of an abdominal mass in neonates

C is inherited as an X-linked recessive trait

D is a recognised complication of maternal rubella infection

E characteristically causes maternal polyhydramnios

Your answers: A.........B.........C.........D.........E.........

9. A single large dose of a suitable antibiotic is appropriate treatment for

A a woman with the acute urethral syndrome but no pyuria

B an asymptomatic non-pregnant woman with bacteriuria

C a urinary tract infection in a male

D a four-year-old girl with her first documented urinary tract infection

E an infected cyst in a polycystic kidney

Your answers: A.........B.........C.........D.........E.........

Answers overleaf

97. B

Most children will have minimal change glomerulopathy and so biopsy is only indicated if proteinuria is non-selective there is no response to steroids. Hypoalbuminaemia and proteinuria reduce the oncotic pressure gradient across the glomerulus and will increase filtration. Both minimal change glomerulopathy and focal segmental glomerulosclerosis may respond to cyclophosphamide in spite of steroid resistance The high serum cholesterol concentration in nephrotic syndrome interferes with the anti-streptolysin O antibody assay.

98. None are correct

Infantile polycystic kidney disease is inherited as an autosomal dominant trait and there is no evidence of its being caused by teratogens or intrauterine infection. It affects both kidney causing bilateral abdominal masses that may result obstructed labour. Congenital hydronephrosis is the most common cause of an abdominal mass in a neonate. As with other causes of intra-uterine renal failure, maternal oligohydramnios is common.

99. B D

The acute urethral syndrome is unlikely to be due to infection with *Chlamydia* or an 'insignificant' number of bacteria in the absence of pyuria. Single dose chemotherapy is the treatment of choice for asymptomatic bacteriuria but has not been fully assessed in pregnancy. Urinary tract infection in male usually reflects an underlying structural or neurological defect for which prolonged administration of antibiotics is indicated An early relapse after single dose chemotherapy identifies children who require further investigation to exclude reflux other urinary tract anomalies. Diffusion of adequate amount of antibiotics to the centre of renal cysts takes several weeks of continuous therapy.

0. Reduced proteinuria in the nephrotic syndrome is recognised following:

A indomethacin

B measles

C renal vein thrombosis

D infusion of salt-poor albumin

E restriction of salt intake

Your answers: A.........B.........C.........D.........E.........

1. In patients with acute renal failure

A eosinophilia and hypocomplementaemia are typical of allergic interstitial nephritis

B non-oliguria indicates a better prognosis

C dopamine typically causes diuresis

D renal obstruction is excluded by polyuria

E aminoglycosides are always contraindicated

Your answers: A.........B.........C.........D.........E.........

2. Renin

A is released from the cells of the macula densa in response to sodium depletion

B release is stimulated by renal sympathetic nervous stimulation

C increases in response to cortical ischaemia

D leads to the production of a plasma borne vasoconstrictor

E leads to an increase in thirst

Your answers: A.........B.........C.........D.........E.........

Answers overleaf

100. A B

Indomethacin reduces proteinuria by inhibiting renal synthes
of vasodilating prostaglandins and so allowing the unoppose
action of angiotensin to reduce renal perfusion. Although vir
infections may exacerbate proteinuria, remission of minim
change glomerulonephritis is well recognised following vir
infections. Indeed, deliberate infection with measles was on
an accepted treatment. Thrombosis of the renal vein is fre
quently locally silent but may present acutely with loin pai
haematuria and increased proteinuria. Salt-poor albumin inf
sions usually increase proteinuria. Low salt diets reduc
oedema but have little effect on proteinuria.

101. B

Acute allergic interstitial nephritis is not characteristical
associated with hypocomplementaemia; a low serum comple
ment and eosinophilia would suggest atheroembolic diseas
Non-oliguric patients usually have less severe renal failur
and have a better prognosis. Although dopamine at a dose
2-5 μg/kg/min may increase renal blood flow this is n
necessarily accompanied by a diuresis. Intermittent or parti
obstruction both cause nephrogenic diabetes insipidus an
may also cause salt wasting. It is worth knowing tha
aminoglycosides may be given in non-toxic doses even t
patients whose renal failure is due to aminoglycoside toxicit
without jeopardising their recovery, although as a general rul
they should be avoided if at all possible.

102. B C D E

Renin is a proteolytic enzyme found in the granular cells of th
juxta-glomerular apparatus and produced in response t
sodium depletion (detected by the cells of the macula dens
or to volume depletion (detected by the atrial and renal capil
ary baroreceptors). Reduced atrial stretch results in increase
renal sympathetic tone and renin release. Renin acts o
angiotensinogen (renin substrate) to produce angiotensin
which is converted to angiotensin II, a potent vasoconstricto
which also stimulates thirst. Redistribution of renal blood flo
away from the outer cortex stimulates renin release, whic
may be of relevance to sodium retention in some diseas
states.

REVISION INDEX